EGO STATES

Theory and Therapy

EGO STATES
THEORY AND THERAPY

John G. Watkins, Ph.D.
and
Helen H. Watkins, M.A.

W. W. NORTON AND COMPANY • New York • London

For information about permission to reproduce selections
from this book, write to
Permissions, W. W. Norton & Company, Inc., 500 Fifth Avenue,
New York, NY 10110.

Library of Congress Cataloging-in-Publication Data

Watkins, John G. (John Goodrich), 1913–
   Ego states : theory and therapy / John G. Watkins and Helen H.
Watkins.
     p.   cm.
   "A Norton professional book"–CIP galley.
   Includes bibliographical references and index.
   ISBN 0-393-70259-6
   1. Dissociative disorders. 2. Ego (Psychology) 3. Hypnotism–
Therapeutic use. I. Watkins, Helen Huth. II. Title.
RC553.D5W38   1997
616.85'23–dc21   97-8401 CIP

W. W. Norton & Company, Inc., 500 Fifth Avenue, New York, N.Y. 10110
http://www.wwnorton.com
W. W. Norton & Company Ltd., 10 Coptic Street, London WC1A 1PU

1 2 3 4 5 6 7 8 9 0

FOREWORD

Ernst Federn

At the 1918 International Congress of Psychoanalysis in Budapest (the first after World War I), Freud presented a lecture about the necessity of utilizing suggestion and hypnotic techniques with psychoanalytic understanding. He found that necessary because society should in the future be able to finance treatment for the masses who suffer psychological problems.

This book, *Ego States: Theory and Therapy*, undertakes to integrate hypnotherapeutic techniques with psychoanalytic concepts in achieving a brief psychotherapy on the basis of Paul Federn's ego psychology, especially on his discovery of the existence of ego states.

Although Freud had started a psychoanalytic ego psychology with his book, *The Ego and the Id* (1923), he did not go further than posing that the psyche of man is divided into an id, an ego, and a superego, with the ego assuming most of the functions of synthesizing and recognizing dangers through anxiety.

While Anna Freud (1946) extended these functions to the mechanisms of defense and Hartmann (1939) to the function of adaptation, Paul Federn discovered the essence of the ego through his work with the mentally ill. This discovery was for a long time neglected by most psychoanalysts, but the authors of this book recognize ego states and work with them with much success in their therapy.

They present Federn's concept of ego states very lucidly and show how they

---

Psychoanalyst Ernst Federn, an Honorary Member of the Vienna Psychoanalytic Society, is the son of Paul Federn, and a distinguished contributor in his own right (see Federn, E., 1960, 1990).   —J.G.W.

must be used in the treatment of multiple personalities and other conditions involving ego disturbances. Employing Federn's concepts of the ego, psychotherapists will secure a theoretical basis for their work, and hypnotherapists can especially profit from such understanding.

CONTENTS

INTRODUCTION

During World War II one of us (JGW), while serving as chief psychologist of a large Army hospital, had referred to him a young lieutenant who suffered from a phobia of the dark. The case was treated hypnoanalytically. It was published in detail (Watkins, J., 1949) and more recently in abbreviated form (Watkins, J., 1992b). The successful resolution of this case involved the discovery that more than one "entity" was involved. At that time I (JGW) would have considered the patient to be a multiple personality. However, the two subpersonalities did not emerge spontaneously, but they could be activated hypnotically. A wide variety of hypnotic, analytic, and projective techniques were employed in understanding them and the interactions which had created a phobia of the dark. The phobia was resolved by psychodynamic insights achieved through hypnoanalytic procedures that have been described in detail elsewhere (Watkins, J., 1992b). As fascinating as these complex interactions were, their most important contribution to the present work was that this was our first direct acquaintance with those covertly segmented personality structures which we now call "ego states."

In the 40 years following World War II I spent much time exploring the modality of hypnosis, both in research and in clinical practice (Watkins, J., 1946, 1947, 1949, 1951, 1954, 1963a, 1963b, 1967, 1971, 1972, 1977, 1978a, 1978b, 1984, 1987, 1989). A personal analysis with training analyst Edoardo Weiss (1960), who had himself been analyzed by Paul Federn and trained by Freud, brought acquaintance with Federn's ego-state theories, which will be described later. This experience further consolidated our understanding of human personality as a multiplicity rather than a unity.

Throughout the 1950s and 1960s I had occasion to treat a number of true multiple personalities, to observe such cases being handled by Bernauer Newton and other colleagues, and to collaborate in preparing reports and audiovisual materials depicting these patients (see Bowers et al., 1971). This experience was very valuable in preparing the ground for an understanding of covert personality entities as compared to true, overt multiple personalities. But the real significance of the "separating defense" as being more broadly based throughout a continuum extending from normal personality structure at one end to severely dissociated personalities at the other end did not emerge until collaboration in the early 1970s with my wife and colleague, Helen H. Watkins (HHW).

Helen, a psychologist in the Counseling Center of the University of Montana, had been treating many normal and neurotic problems among college students. As a skilled hypnotherapist she kept seeing these covert alters appearing in her clients, creating intrapersonal conflicts and requiring understanding for successful therapy. I, too, began to employ hypnoanalytic techniques with covert personality segments as well as with the entire individual and found both my clinical understanding and therapeutic success enhanced. Furthermore, the theories of Paul Federn (1952) and Edoardo Weiss (1960) to which I had been exposed some two decades earlier seemed very relevant to these present cases.

During these years, as professor and director of training for the University of Montana's clinical psychology program, much time was spent teaching and supervising students and working with them on masters theses and doctoral dissertations, some related to ego states (Douglass & Watkins, 1994; Eibl-mayr, 1987; Hartman, W., 1995).

Although Helen was engaged primarily during these years with general clinical practice, I tended to restrict my cases more to true multiple personalities. The need to understand and deal with both overt and covert personality segments impelled us to confer frequently, sometimes sitting in on each other's treatment sessions, and develop together a coherent ego-state theory and therapy system.

Helen seemed to possess a kind of "third ear" sensitivity (Reik, 1948). So many times she would zero-in on the behavior of covert personality segments and devise innovative therapeutic strategies for dealing with them. We would combine these with earlier hypnoanalytic procedures that I had developed, such as abreactions (Watkins, J., 1949), projective techniques (1952), and the affect bridge (1971).

My own need was to investigate the nature of these "ego states" and to develop a theoretical rationale for understanding them. Accordingly, we collaborated in experimental studies (Watkins & Watkins, 1979–80, 1980) and constantly discussed and argued the theory that began unfolding (Watkins, H., 1993). Helen provided increasing bits of data and case material from her practice, and I kept trying to make more theoretical meaning out of all these. We began a series of workshop presentations (see Steckler, 1989) and publications (Watkins & Watkins, 1979, 1981, 1982, 1984, 1986, 1988, 1990a, 1990b, 1991, 1992, 1993a, 1996a). Friends and colleagues with whom we discussed our ideas picked up the ego state concepts and proceeded to test them out in practice and to develop their own lines of investigation and theories (Beahrs, 1982, 1986; Edelstien, 1982; Frederick, 1993, Frederick & McNeal, 1993; Frederick & Phillips, 1995; Newey, 1986; Phillips, 1993; Phillips & Frederick, 1995; Torem, 1987, 1989, 1993).

Independently, Hilgard (1977, 1986) presented studies on "the hidden observer" phenomenon, which further demonstrated the factor of "co-consciousness" (Beahrs, 1983) in personality functioning. The term Hilgard used, "cognitive structural systems," seemed to include the same entities that we had called "ego states," and with which we had worked therapeutically (Watkins & Watkins 1979–80, 1980). The studies by Bower (1981) and associates (1978) on mood and memory also tended to reinforce the ego state concept.

Within the past two decades there has been a revival of interest in multiple personalities and the entire field of dissociation. Led by such investigators as Bliss (1986), Boor and Coons (1983), Braun (1984), Caul (1988), Coons (1988, 1993), Fine (1989, 1993), Greaves (1988), Kluft (1987, 1988, 1993), Kluft and Fine (1993), Loewenstein (1991), Putnam (1985, 1989, 1991), Ross (1989, 1991) and others, this diagnosis has gained increased study and respectability. The *DSM-IV* of the American Psychiatric Association (APA, 1994) has devoted much space to a refined definition and criteria for dissociative conditions. Multiple personality disorder (MPD) has been renamed dissociative identity disorder (DID).

A new scientific organization, the International Society for the Study of Dissociation, has been formed. Its membership currently numbers over 3000 mental health professionals, and its professional journal, *Dissociation*, regularly publishes a wealth of new studies in the field. Furthermore, hypnosis itself is now being regarded as primarily a form of dissociation rather than merely suggestion (Hilgard, 1986).

The literature on diagnosis and treatment of multiple personality today is filled with increasing use of the term "ego states" and recognition of the existence of covert personality segments as well as the more overt ones found in true multiples (Brown & Fromm, 1986; Gruenwald, 1986; Ramonth, 1985). Accordingly, it seems to us that a theory linking normal personality functioning with its extremes of dissociation as found in multiple personalities, amnesias, and fugue states needs exposition at the present time. From such a rationale, perhaps better ways of treating true multiples could be developed as well as dealing with the more normal and neurotic disorders that result from lesser forms of separation.

Instead of regarding multiplicity as some extreme and radical division of human personality functioning, it could be seen, when pathological, as simply the result of excess in adaptational and defense processes used by all individuals for protection and survival. This concept has been proposed and extensively elaborated by Beahrs (1982, 1986).

In this work we hope to bring together our experience, research, and clinical practice with that of others into a coherent approach that we have termed "ego state therapy." We are indebted to such earlier thinkers as Janet (1907), Federn (1952), and Weiss (1960), and to numerous psychoanalytic theorists and practitioners. We realize that our theories here also touch on those of the object-relations analysts, such as Fairbairn (1963), Guntrip (1968, 1971), Jacobson (1964), Kernberg (1976), Kohut (1978), Mahler (1978), Winnicott (1971), and others.

Psychotherapists are currently confronted with a serious problem. Psychodynamic therapies (such as psychoanalysis) have usually required many sessions, commonly spread over months and years. Today, insurance companies and other third-party payers will not fund such lengthy treatments. They demand brief and "efficient" therapies. Therapists who practice approaches (such as psychoanalysis), that require several sessions a week over many months, are faced with a severe economic crisis (Goldberg, 1996). Hypnoanalysis (Fromm & Nash, 1997; Watkins, J., 1992a, 1992b) has demonstrated that it can significantly shorten the time for "analytic" treatment. Intensive ego state therapy, which is an extension of hypnoanalysis, may offer an effective and even briefer approach, which within 8–12 hours (according to our follow-up research studies–see chapter 13) often achieves permanent, structural personality changes, including the resolution of life-long disorders.

The science of psychology and the therapeutic treatment of human personality disturbances is a constantly evolving field. In fact, the advance is so rapid that it is virtually impossible for any single individual to keep fully abreast of new developments in even a small facet of knowledge–such as dissociation. We therefore offer our contribution here with the full recognition that we will have undoubtedly failed to become acquainted with and give recognition to many other thinkers, researchers, and practitioners who have been wrestling with these same concepts earlier and contemporarily, perhaps with a different terminology.

Today's pronounced information overload and communication gap leads presumed innovators to reinvent the wheel. We are also aware that the true inventor borrows from the widest number of sources. So it is with a genuine sense of humility that we present the product of our joint research, theoretical conceptualizations, clinical practice, plus the stimulation of others. We do realize that ego state therapy has attracted the attention of colleagues and other contributors who are now developing the field further, and we look forward to continued advances in this approach.

Since our current stage and development of ego state therapy is the culmination of many earlier studies, which we have published individually and jointly, we will often make reference to these for the benefit of those readers who wish a more complete presentation of a particular theoretical point or clinical technique.

We recognize that in a short time our views may be out of date. But we shall be content if in some way they add to the growing understanding of human personality functioning, both adaptive and maladaptive.

John G. Watkins

1

PERSONALITY AND ITS DEVELOPMENT

Personality is a very difficult concept to define. Yet the term is widely used and when spoken transmits meaning between people. If we say, "She has a sparkling personality," we picture her as pleasantly intriguing. It also suggests that in a social situation we expect her to be quite popular and sought after. On the other hand, if we describe a man as having "a rotten personality," we anticipate that he would tend to alienate others and would not likely make a good salesman. The word conveys many meanings in common language, even though behavioral scientists have a most difficult time pinning down a formal definition that includes all aspects of personality while excluding other psychological manifestations. The essence here seems to be those characteristics of a person whose behavioral manifestations are evaluated and reacted to by others.

Many scholars have attempted the difficult task of describing personality, seeking its essential dimensions, and developing a rationale to explain its development and functioning. These include Adler (1963), Allport (1955), Freud (1938), Fromm, Erik (1964), Fromm, Erika (1977), Horney (1950), Jung (1934, 1969), Maslow (1968), May (1980), Piaget (1963, 1966), Rank (1950), Rogers (1980), Sullivan (1980), to name but a few, plus the contributions of the object-relations theorists, such as Kernberg (1976), Kohut (1977), Mahler (1978), Winnicott (1965), and many others. The innovators and contributors to personality theory are legion, and we shall make no attempt here to review their publications or even to recognize all.

This book is another such effort to understand "personality." Accordingly, we will try to indicate those earlier writers whose contributions are related to ego state theory or have directly influenced it.

When speaking of ego state theory, what do we mean by the word *theory?*

1

A theory is simply a way of looking at a set of data. Hall & Lindzey (1985) have called attention to the fact that a theory is not necessarily true or false. Rather it should be considered as useful or not useful, depending on whether its predictions are borne out and whether events can be controlled when it is applied to observations. A theory also should generate research hypotheses while suggesting new and as yet unobserved relations. Its purpose is to make prior assumptions explicit.

Theories have been developed to try and answer man's never-ending search to understand himself and his fellow beings and to provide a sensible rationale for dealing with them. Some theories have been developed from clinical studies of human behavior, others from laboratory research, and still others from philosophical speculation about the nature of man. Ours has drawn on all three.

But what constitutes a good personality theory? R. Ewen (1980) has suggested that a good theory should provide convenient descriptions of the relevant behavior, offer a framework for organizing data, and focus attention on matters of greater importance. He holds also that it should explain the phenomena under study and offer answers to questions about individual differences and why some persons become more affected than others. Furthermore, a good theory should generate predictions that lead to practical applications that facilitate change and control of the environment.

As new data concerning human behavior becomes available, from both experimental research and clinical experience with patients, new theories will be developed that hopefully will better explain the observed phenomena and make more precise the therapeutic manipulations to be used in ameliorating pathology.

Personality theory-makers often borrow concepts from earlier theoreticians as well as from more recent observations and research. The quest is for a more meaningful rationale and more valid interventions. One should not put forward a "new" theory that is merely a rehash of concepts already published without giving credit to its earlier promulgators. It is easy to do this since no one person can read all that has been written in the personality field, and hence, through unawareness of a previous formulation, may simply repeat the same cognitive processes by which the theory was first devised.

But all theories are necessarily incomplete. Present-day scientists may start with a known theory, alter its definitions, add to its scope, and render it more applicable, hence improving it. This does not subtract from the credit due its earlier developers. Through all ages human knowledge and understanding advances. It becomes both more complex and more meaningful but is couched in the language of the day.

The ego state theory we will propose here is such an endeavor. It has drawn its sources from many previous theories. However, it has also been built on dissatisfaction with those formulations. These earlier concepts were either not made fully meaningful or they were incomplete and did not adequately describe and explain the phenomena we have observed in our clinical practice. Furthermore, many of them, although beautiful edifices of cognition, did not translate their conclusions into practical applications. Abstraction is often piled on abstraction, and from these many corollaries are spun. There is a paucity of specific, objective case material to illustrate a point; the theorist assumes that his terms are understood by the reader. We have found this true of so many personality theories. They did not help us to understand and treat our patients better. They also provided little technology that would tell us just what to do, what not to do, and how to do it when we practiced therapy with physically present, live patients. Thus they failed to meet many of the criteria of a "good" theory as delineated by Ewen.

Since ego state theory has evolved from concepts proposed by earlier contributors, it is appropriate that we review several to whom we owe the greatest debt.

Ellenberger (1970) noted that St. Augustine in his "Confessions" pondered whether personality was a unity, and that "divided personality" was known by the end of the eighteenth century. By 1880 it was a matter of discussion by both psychiatrists and philosophers. While dissociation had been observed by many of the early workers with hypnosis, Janet (1907, 1925) described this phenomenon and "unconscious" processes in various patients, apparently before Freud.

Janet noted that in the development of language an action gradually became separated from the verbalized sound that originally accompanied the action and later came to cue it. Hence, language itself became "dissociated" from its external behavior, permitting an individual to "exist" at times in an internal world differentiated from "real," external existence. This kind of dissociation is normal in all people.

Janet observed that the quantum of energy utilized in the controlling processes, for example, thinking, verbalizing, is much less than that expended in the controlled processes of physical behavior. From an evolutionary standpoint it is more economic when behaviors can be tried out mentally before being carried out physically. This separating results in greatly increased potential for efficient behavior. Differentiation is therefore a building process fundamental to the evolutional development of intelligent-behaving humans. It is economical to control large expenditures of behavior with the expenditure of much smaller quantums of energy by higher level, controlling (thought) processes. It also increases the likelihood that once the behavioral actions are initiated, maladaptive results will be minimized and successful outcomes enhanced. Organisms (such as homo sapiens) that developed this differentiating ability became the surviving and ruling species.

Janet also reduced psychological processes to the flowing and ebbing of higher and lower level energies. The concept of mental energies, of course, has also held a central position in the theories of both Jung (1969) and Freud (1938). Energy conceptions became an integral part of the theories of Paul Federn (1952). His views especially influenced our own ego state theories and will be discussed later in more detail.

Janet held that a system of ideas became dissociated from the main personality and could exist as a subconscious personality. This personality was generally unconscious to the individual but could become conscious through hypnosis. This definition of subconscious personality is almost identical with that of ego state, which we will describe later.

However, the early workers with dissociation gathered their data primarily from the study of hysterical or psychopathologically ill patients. Accordingly, dissociation came to be regarded as an abnormal condition, found primarily in mentally ill individuals. While the studies in ego states encompass these severe forms of dissociation observed in abnormal behavior, many of our findings have been drawn from the study or treatment of individuals with normal problems (such as overweight, poor study habits, or smoking), as well as with neurotic and psychophysiological conditions.

A great deal of controversy has occurred over the extent to which subconscious personalities interfere with the normal functioning of the major personality. Thus Nadon, D'Eon, McKonkey, Laurance, & Campbell (1988) reported that the activity of the secondary intelligence tended to inhibit the flow of thought of the principal intelligence.

Other investigators attempted to discredit the concept of dissociation with studies demonstrating that the interference should be complete or the concept should be discarded. Hilgard (1986, 1987) has reviewed these studies at length and noted (1986, p. 12), "The originators of the concept (dissociation)[1] held no such extreme positions," and considered it sensible to accept that interference can be partial. This is precisely the position we take here, except to suggest that a better term than "interference" might be "influence." This influence by subentities may modify or even facilitate the functioning of the primary personality, as well as interfere with it. Ego state theory also presents a rationale to account for different degrees of interference or influence, and why this process may be more or less conscious.

Jung's system of analytical psychology (1969) is a very complex set of contributions to the understanding of personality functioning, and many of his concepts were forerunners of those to be elaborated here (and of Paul Federn, whose psychology will be described in chapter 2). Although Jung based his theories primarily on clinical practice, there is a certain mysticism in them that makes it difficult for more "objective" scientists to appreciate their significance. We will consider here only those concepts of Jung that bear more directly on the development of ego state theory.

Both of the major contributions of Federn on which ego state theory is based were mentioned earlier by Jung: The concept of psychic energy and the belief that personality is a multiplicity and not just a unity. Jung viewed the psyche as having different components capable of gravitating between the conscious and the unconscious, a position elaborated by Beahrs (1986). Jung posited the existence within the personality of "complexes," a group of unconscious ideas that clustered together. He also held that a person does not have a complex. The complex has *him*. This concept seems to be very close to Federn's ego states, and to our position of the executive ego state, that is, the self in the now, which is especially manifested in multiple personalities. Jung also described archetypes, permanent covert structures within the collective or racial unconscious. While ego state therapy does not posit such entities, Jung's concept of the multiplicity inherent in human experience and behavior is basic to our theory.

The concept of psychic energies is in accord with Freud's libido and with Federn's ego and object cathexes, although defined differently and qualitatively different in function. Sullivan (1980) also considered the human being as an energy system. Accordingly, this concept has been voiced by many earlier contributors. However, in ego state theory we will see efforts to apply this concept more specifically to the understanding of mental disorders and their treatment.

Our ego state theory has also been influenced by recent findings, such as Hilgard's neo-dissociation theory of hypnosis and his studies with the "hidden observer" phenomenon (1977, 1986; see also Nadon et al., 1988). However, our first formulations of ego state theory began in the early 1970s. The work by Braun (1986), Coons (1984), Kluft (1987), Kluft and Fine (1993), Putnam (1986), Ross (1989), and other recent workers in the field of dissociation has contributed to the modifications and development of both theory and practice in ego state psychology.

We have been presenting this theory and practice in a number of workshops (see Steckler, 1989) and have found substantial enthusiasm for these concepts, and clinicians have written us about their success in treating patients from the viewpoint of personality as a multiplicity. We hope further research will strengthen those concepts which have emerged from the practice area.

No "depth" psychology or analytic treatment can be proposed without recognition of the monumental influence of Freud and his followers. His

studies of unconscious processes and the defense mechanisms, especially repression, are fundamental in any investigation of human motivation–and
have even influenced hypnosis, which he originally tried and discarded. We
acknowledge our immense debt to the many discoveries and developments of
psychoanalysis and the dozens of ways in which psychoanalytic thinking has
influenced both our theory and therapy. In fact, it was through the process
of personal analysis and subsequent training from Edoardo Weiss (a Freudian
analyst), plus hypnotherapy research and practice, that one of us (JGW)
developed his original interest in the exploration of unconscious processes.

In presenting ego state theory and therapy here, we will endeavor:

- to show the sources from which it was developed,
- to give credit to those earlier thinkers who first proposed concepts which we will use,
- to demonstrate wherein we found their theoretical contribution incomplete or inadequate to explain the behavioral and experiential phenomena,
- to indicate just where we agree and where we differ from the original conceptions of Federn,
- to propose such modifications as we believe will make these phenomena more understandable, and
- to present therapeutic procedures based on that understanding, tested on our patients, and which we have found to be effective in their treatment.

Concepts used will be defined and explained and examples given to assure
that the reader will give to them the same meanings we do. In some cases the
sense in which we use a term will not be the same as that of other theoreticians or practitioners. The effort will be to try and make ego state theory
understandable, whether or not it ultimately proves to be valid.

Ego state therapy, though an analytic treatment, differs in significant ways
(both conceptually and in techniques of practice) from classical psychoanalysis. Accordingly, we turn to the theories of Paul Federn (1943, 1947a, 1947b,
1952), a long and close associate of Freud, and to the expositions of these by
Federn's analysand and protege, Edoardo Weiss, as the next great source of
influence from which ego state theory and practice has developed.

Federn proposed a two-energy theory to explain many psychological phenomena for which Freud's one-energy theory (libido) could not adequately
account. Weiss (1960, 1966) elaborated it further, based on his psychoanalysis of clinical cases. We have modified it still further from the influence of

experimental as well as clinical data. It is our belief that Federn's concepts can be applied more widely to the treatment of dissociation and a broad spectrum of other psychogenic disorders as well as normal problems of adjustment, conditions to which neither Federn nor Weiss paid much attention. Ego state therapy is accordingly a set of therapeutic tactics and strategies based on modifications of their theories and as influenced by the other writers mentioned in this chapter. It involves a somewhat different way of viewing normal personality, its development, its pathologies, and especially the concept of what constitutes "the self."

2

ENERGIES AND PERSONALITY FUNCTIONING

We experience our existence because of two dichotomous personality functions: conscious-unconscious and subject-object. Let us define what we mean by each term and then apply to it an "energy theory" that may provide a rationale to account for its manifestations and changes.

Conscious-Unconscious

Just what do we mean when we say we are *conscious* of something? Webster's dictionary defines conscious as follows: "aware, to know with, having a feeling or knowledge (of one's) sensations, feelings, etc., or external things; aware of oneself as a thinking being; knowing what one is doing and why, known to, or felt by oneself as conscious guilt."

But all these definitions hinge on what is meant by "self." As we experience ourselves what is meant seems quite clear, but when we begin to study dissociations, ego states, and multiple personalities the distinction becomes unclear.

In another work (Watkins, J., 1978a) it was proposed that "existence is impact," impact between an entity invested with ego or self-energy and an element "cathected" with an object or non-self-energy. According to this conception, for consciousness to take place there would have to be two parties involved, that which is doing the "consciousnessing" and that which is being "consciousnessed." As we consider further the sectioning of the self into ego states or multiple personality alters, we must recognize that simply to claim that an individual was conscious without specifying just what within the person was conscious is an inadequate statement.

If a hypnotic subject's hand is made to wag up and down posthypnotically,

8

is the subject conscious of it? Certainly he observes it wagging up and down, but at the present he does not regard it as a part of himself. He is not conscious of *why* it is wagging up and down. He is not conscious that *he* is doing it. He perceives the experience as if he were observing somebody else's hand moving up and down. That a behavioral movement in one's body is overt and can be observed by one's self or others does not necessarily make it conscious.

We would also not regard the sleepwalker as being conscious of his behavior, although probably if we were to hypnotize him later and inquire within we could activate an ego state, a covert part of him, which might say to us, "Yes. I went walking last night, but he (the normally overt personality) didn't know about it." Shall we say then that the hypnotically activated ego state was conscious of the behavior although the main personality was not?

Consider a dialogue between two alters in a multiple. When alter A speaks, he is conscious that he is doing the speaking. And when alter B replies, he is consciously hearing the speech of the other, but is not aware that he, himself,[1] is speaking. Would we then say that the "person" is conscious of what is transpiring? Obviously an action or a communication may be overt and observable to others and still be conscious to only one part of one's personality.

Yet we may be fully aware of a mental activity within our self, such as a dream, and there is no overt behavior observable to others. Furthermore, we "see" the dream images and sometimes participate in aspects of them with a feeling of selfness, and we can remember them on awakening and describe our behavior in the dream, yet we do not consider a dream as being conscious behavior.

People may be well aware of their actions, yet not be consciously aware of the *unconscious* motivations that initiate them. It is obvious that when we label any thought or action as conscious we need to specify just what it was that was conscious and to whom. Because an individual is aware of a mental process, thought, or perception emanating from within his brain or carried out by his body does not make it conscious. But in most cases if we explore throughout the whole personality, perhaps by hypnosis, we will discover that the mental process, or action, was conscious to some part of the entire personality, a part that can tell us, "Yes, I did it, and I intended to do it." And although it was conscious to one or more segments within the person, it was unconscious to others. That is because persons are multiplicities, not unities.

An act may also be conscious to an individual, and he is held accountable for it, even though we may say, "He is not conscious of its effect on others." This poses a tremendous problem in courts of law. At what point is an action conscious, and just when should the individual be held accountable for it?

This legal dilemma is discussed elsewhere as applied to specific forensic cases (see Watkins, J., 1976, 1978b, 1989, 1993a).

Subject-Object

Human existence requires another dimension to describe it besides conscious or unconscious. I may be conscious of a hallucination, but I am not conscious that it is "my" thought. Consciously I experience it as a perception of stimuli coming from an outside object. My experience is that this object exists outside of me. I am not conscious of the location of the origin of this experience. Likewise, I may claim credit for a new idea which is merely the repetition of a perception I received from another person. In this case I am conscious of the perception, but impute its origin to a creative process within my own self. It is clear that merely being conscious of an item (perception or thought) does not adequately depict my true "existence." Some other process is involved. This process is the phenomenon of *subject-object*.

Subject means not only something that is experienced, but something that is also experienced as a stimulus whose origin lies within my own self, within me. If I move a hand up and down, it is I, *my self*, that is moving it. If I am conscious of a thought, it is experienced as stemming from me. It is my thought. From this perspective my existence is defined by the experience of my self as being the originating locus for whatever stimulus is evoking my consciousness, my awareness of it.

Sometimes my existential experience involves both internal and external stimuli, as for example, when I am reading a book of fiction. The little black marks on the page outside me (objects) are initiating in me patterns of stimuli which I usually experience when observing something on the outside, a play or activities of other people. Yet the exact content of the images in which I experience the drama of the story is being elaborated by inside stimuli. The existence experience at that time is both subject and object.

This dual nature of the image is quite clear if a person reads the following sentence in a novel: "The girl ran down the street." If asked to describe one's internal picturing, an individual may state that the girl is a blonde, while another might point out that she is a brunette. The image of "girl running" is initiated by the external stimulus of the printed word, and hence, is object. Yet, its elaboration, namely that the girl is blonde, stems from an internal and personal stimulus and is therefore subject.

The contamination of witness memories by internal stimuli, not stemming from the direct observation of an external event, is a considerable problem in forensic cases. The extent of such interference and its effect on the credibility of eyewitness testimony, both in and out of hypnosis, has had considerable study (Hilgard & Loftus, 1979; Loftus, 1979; Watkins, J., 1989, 1993a).

The ability for a psychological item to be either subject or object is most observable in dreams. Consider the following:

- "I dreamed I saw a man beating a small boy, but it didn't bother me. I didn't recognize either of them." In this case both the man and the boy are perceived as object, not part of the self. The dreamer is not "bothered."

- "I dreamed I saw a man beating a small boy, and I felt very sorry for the boy. He didn't deserve it." Here, the dreamer still treats both the man and the boy as objects, but he is beginning to resonate with the boy, suggesting that he is close to identifying himself with the boy. He "feels with" the boy, a kind of "affective identification."

- "I dreamed I saw a man beating a boy who looked like me." The dreamer lacks an affective identification, but shows a cognitive and visual kinship. The boy is still object.

- "I dreamed my father was giving me a licking, and it sure hurt." Identification with the boy is complete. The boy has now become subject, part of the dreamer's self (he calls it "me") while the father is still viewed as object.

- "I dreamed I was spanking my son because he had behaved badly." In this case the dreamer now identifies with the man and views the boy as object. He has identified with his father, who is now experienced as subject, part of his own self.

It is clear that all of these dream experiences are from the same original psychological thoughts. They are the same dream, but experienced in different ways depending on which elements are made subject and which object by the dreamer.

An internal stimulus may be experienced dream-wise by one segment of a personality as subject and at the same time by another segment as object. A multiple personality by the name of Jane described a dream she had during which she was standing beside her boyfriend in a grocery store when a masked man broke in and fired a shot. She screamed and awakened in a panic. Later in the therapeutic session an underlying alter, Lynne, emerged and spontaneously described a dream she had in which she was walking along a sidewalk in front of a supermarket when a black car stopped. A masked man with a gun got out and ran into the store. Then she heard a shot and a scream. Notice that for Jane her experience was that "I screamed," hence the scream was a subject experience. Lynne, a different ego state within the same body, experienced the same stimulus as object, "I heard a scream."

Subjective experiences are not directly amenable to verification as are objective experiences. That is why behaviorists attempted to rule them out as sources of scientific data. According to behaviorists only observations that can be independently perceived by outside observers should be permitted in a methodologically sound psychology. This attitude resulted in such jokes as the behaviorist who remarked to a colleague one morning, "You are fine. How am I?"

While we must agree that reports of subject experiences are more at risk for misperception and contamination than object perceptions, nevertheless we cannot ignore such data without eliminating a large part and perhaps the most significant aspect of human existence. We can make evaluations of subject experiences by verbal report (introspections[2]) and by indirect objective observations of behaviors commonly related to them, for example, the unplanned "ouch" shouted by an individual being stimulated in a way that creates pain.

Not only must we pay attention to subject experiences as well as object ones, but we also need to be able to label each, to ascertain how much of an experience stems from subject, hence internal, stimuli, and how much from outside, object stimuli. Failure to do this is the source of many false conclusions from psychological experiments. The internal interpretation of what is happening or what a person is doing may be the really significant finding in a study.

An older boy, to prove how dumb his little brother was, would show the younger one a nickel and a dime before friends and ask him to take his pick. The little fellow invariably picked the nickel, much to the amusement of the group, who thought he was deciding on the basis of its size. When asked later, the young one said, "I take the nickel because I can make more money that way. If I ever took the dime he wouldn't do it again." Objective observation of behavior alone can often be misleading.

As we shall be constantly noting in this book, the distinction between subject and object becomes especially important when using hypnosis, when treating multiple personalities, or when doing ego state therapy. Our understanding of any mental phenomenon will be very faulty unless we always consider it from both the subject and the object perspectives.

With a fairly clear conception of what is meant by the terms *conscious, unconscious, subject,* and *object* we can now proceed to an energy theory proposed by Paul Federn (1952) that provides a rationale for these terms—even though Federn himself and his protege, Edoardo Weiss (1960), never really applied their conceptions to many phenomena with which we will be much concerned here, such as hypnosis and multiple personality.

The Ego Psychology of Paul Federn

Federn (1928, 1932, 1943, 1947a, 1947b, 1952) was one of the earliest and most faithful of Freud's disciples, maintaining a continuous relationship from 1903 until Freud's death in 1939. He is described as having a great breadth of scientific and literary interests and being a very sensitive and creative therapist. He was also a prolific writer and developed many creative modifications of psychoanalysis, especially in ego psychology. Unfortunately, his views were not widely understood by other analysts. Federn was a modest man and had a tendency to subordinate his own innovations to those of Freud. During the intense theoretical debates within the Vienna Psychoanalytic Society, his was the more mild and moderating voice.

Following the Nazi occupation of Austria in 1938, Federn moved to New York. He suffered from depressive moods and was preoccupied with the persistent idea that he would eventually end his own life–which he did after falling victim to an untreatable cancer. He outlived Freud by eleven years.

Federn's views on the ego significantly differed from those of the other ego psychologists within the psychoanalytic movement, such as Hartmann (1939), Kris (1951), Rappaport (1967), and those of the much later object-relation theorists, including Guntrip (1971), Jacobson (1954), Kernberg (1976), Kohut (1977), and Winnicott (1965). In fact, many of the contributions of these later workers, especially in regard to ego states, had been anticipated by Federn, although in a somewhat different terminology which was not well understood by his colleagues. This was partly due to the style of his writings. His theoretical conceptions, even when translated into English from the German scientific idiom, are rather complex and difficult to comprehend. We will attempt here to describe only those parts of them that are relevant to the theory and practice of ego state therapy. A somewhat more detailed explication has been published by JGW in his book *The Therapeutic Self* (1978a).

FEDERN'S TWO-ENERGY THEORY

Freud developed his *libido* theory (1905, 1922) to explain flows of energy that activated various psychological processes. However, many difficulties arose with libido theory, partly because Freud (1923) described this energy as erotic in nature. Other writers (Jung, 1969) began to use the term to represent a kind of "psychic" or life energy, and the word developed multiple meanings. Freud used the word *cathexis* with libido to indicate a charge of energy that activated a process. Thus, when the image of an another individual was "cathected with libido" this meant that it was invested with an erotic energy, making the individual a love object. The analogy might be made of turning a flashlight in a dark room onto another person. That person would now stand out from other aspects of the environment. Hence, libido was not only an erotic energy but also an object energy, since objects so cathected became energized and important, but external to the self.

Freud (1914) explained narcissism as the redirecting by the individual of this libidinal energy back onto the ego. He then called it *ego-libido*. However, it was the same energy, only its direction had changed from outward to inward.

Federn felt that a single kind of energy, libido, could not explain all the ramifications and decided that ego-libido was not merely the same energy with a redirected objective, but an entirely *different kind* of energy from ordinary libido, qualitatively speaking. He gradually dropped the term "libido" and more frequently referred to two different types of energies: *object cathexis* and *ego cathexis*.

Federn did not denote either of these cathexes as being sexual in nature, even though his object cathexis was similar to Freud's libido. The great difference lay in his conception that when a mental process was invested with object cathexis, that energy by its very investment turned the element into an object. Thus, if a perception of another person was sensed, recorded, and invested with object cathexis, and if it was retained more or less permanently, it became an internal object, an *introject* or *object representation*.

The quantity of object cathexis with which it was invested determined how important an object it was. For example, object cathexis might be compared to the electricity switched into a motor—the greater the amount, the more power and speed the motor can develop. Cathexis, a quantum of energy, like the electricity in a motor, provides the power that activates a psychological process. If it is object cathected, then the representation is perceived by the individual as an object, not as a part of the self. Object cathexis is an inorganic, "it" energy, which by its investment assures that the invested element or any other so-cathected psychological process will be experienced as "not-me." If the internal image of my brother is object cathected, then I experience him as a perception. If an image of my brother is invested with ego-cathexis, then I would experience it as my thought about my brother. Thus, whether a representation becomes object or subject depends on the kind of energy cathecting it.

Federn conceptualized ego cathexis as being the energy of selfness, and any item so invested was experienced as being within one's self, as a part of "the me." Extended still further, ego cathexis is not only the energy of the self, it *is* the self. Self is an energy, not a content, an energy that has only one characteristic, *the feeling of selfness.* Federn (1952, p. 62) further characterized this "ego feeling" as "the residual experience which persists after the subtraction of all ideational contents."

This energy, when it "cathects" or is extended over any psychological or physiological element of the person, provides a "feeling of unity, in continuity, contiguity and causality in the experiences of the individual." Moreover, Federn (1952, p. 185) stated, "I conceive of the ego not merely as the sum of all functions but as the cathexis (energy) which unites the aggregate into a new mental entity.

When a part of my body, such as my arm, is ego-cathected, then I experience it as "my arm." If it is a thought so energized, then I experience it as "my thought." Any physical or mental element becomes part of "me" if and when it is invested with ego cathexis.

The essential concept in whether any part of the body or mind is experienced as "me" or "not-me" is determined by the nature or kind of energy with which it is invested. If the activating energy is object cathexis, then it is experienced as an object, not-me. If its activating energy is ego cathexis, then it is experienced as subject, me, my self. This is not to be confused with conscious or unconscious, since processes within the ego (e.g., defense mechanisms) can be unconscious, and internal objects (introjects) can also be unconscious. As Federn (1952, p. 212) put it, "It would be simple to say that the ego feeling is identical with consciousness, yet there are ego states which are not conscious because they are repressed, and there are conscious object-representations which do not belong to the ego."

By positing a two-energy system, Federn provides a rationale to explain many psychological processes, which cannot be satisfactorily accounted for by a one-energy (libido) system. For example, if a thought of my dead mother reaches consciousness, but is activated with object cathexis, I will experience it as a perception of my dead mother. I will "see" her. And if I report this perception as real, others will say I am psychotic and hallucinating.

Some years ago I was trying to explain the mechanism of projection to a paranoid patient (usually a futile task as most clinicians know). To my surprise he smiled and said, "Well doctor, if you're trying to tell me that those men who persecuted me were a product of my own imagination, you don't have to. I arrived at that conclusion myself over the weekend." In utter amazement I spent some time evaluating him before accepting that somehow, for reasons unknown to me, his delusions and hallucinations had disappeared. His own unconscious hatreds externalized into a perception of "men out there" who were persecuting him, had been decathected of object energy, and were now energized with ego-cathexis. He experienced them as his thoughts and not his perceptions. A one-energy system would not give us as adequate an explanatory rationale, even though psychodynamically we are still unaware of just what caused this energy shift.

Psychologists and psychoanalysts frequently confuse subject and object. Thus, an introject is supposed to be an internal object. Yet analytic writers portray a patient as "introjecting" another person and then describe that individual as acting and talking like the other person. The image of the other, when internalized, is at first invested with object cathexis. That is why it is an internal object. An introject is like a stone in the stomach, within the self but not part of it, ingested but not digested. For the individual to act and talk spontaneously like the other, the object cathexis must be withdrawn and the image ego cathected. In object-relations theory we would say that an *object representation* has been changed into a *self representation*. Then we no longer have an introject; we have an identification. The internalized image has become part of "the me."

For example, a small boy may imitate the behavior of his father, swinging his arms as he strides along. This action is at first an introject, a movement that is simply an internal representation of his father, copied but not a part of his own self. However, in the course of time it may become automatic with him. The movement has become egotized, that is, invested with ego cathexis. It is now part of his own self. The neighbors watch him striding beside his father, both swinging their arms, and remark, "He sure is a chip off the old block." Psychologically we say (at least in this respect), "He has identified with his father." An identification with a previously introjected other may be minimal or significant, depending on how much of the other's physical attributes and/or psychological behavior is taken over.

In another writing (Watkins, J., 1978a) it was suggested that since an introject is the result of the process of introjection, a new term is needed to distinguish between the process of identification and the result of that process. We originally considered using the word "identification" when referring to the process, and the term "identofact" to indicate the internal, ego-cathected image that has been created by identification. The boy described above has changed the introject (an object representation) of his father into an identofact (a self representation). This distinction between what is subject (ego-cathected) and what is not-self (object-cathected) in physical and psychological processes is crucial, and the movement from one to the other is fundamental to the practice of ego state therapy, as well as many other treatment approaches.[3]

THE SELF

Philosophers, psychologists, and psychoanalytic theorists have wrestled with the concept of self. Erik Homberger Erikson, a student of Federn's, sought his own identity in a classic, searching inquiry (1968), which was obviously influenced by Federn's concepts, but reverted more to a re-examination of Freud's ideas. And Hartmann (1964) was apparently the analyst who coined the terms "ego or self representation" and "object representation" as psychic structures that were activated when energized with "libido," terms in much current usage by object relations (Buckley, 1986) and self psychology theorists (Goldberg, 1991). In these one-energy theories, the "selfness" inheres in the mental structures established, not in the kind or "quality" of the activating energy—as in Federn's views.

THE EGO BOUNDARY

The boundaries between the core ego, the various ego states, and the external world constituted the sense organs of the self, permitting one to discriminate between external and internal reality. These boundaries are flexible, expanding and contracting. If an item contacts the external face of a boundary (that which faces the external world), the person can distinguish that item as real. If it contacts the internal boundary, then it is sensed as emanating from one's self.

CONSCIOUSNESS

Federn originally accepted Freud's tripartite division of the personality into id, ego, and super-ego. However, he apparently did not try to explain why something should be conscious or unconscious. It is interesting to extend his two-energy theory and attempt a rationale for consciousness.

Let us think of experiential existence as being the impact of object on subject, of a not-me on the self. The impact of light from an external source on the retina initiates the experience of vision. Yet the impact must be of a certain magnitude for this to take place. If the light is too faint or the retina too weak, then the object will not be seen. Translating this into Federn's two-energy system, an object-cathected stimulus must strike an ego-cathected receptor within an individual for him to perceive it; but if the magnitude of the impact is below a minimal threshold, then he is not aware of it. The stimulus and ego-cathected ego boundaries are not strong enough to evoke the experience we call conscious. However, such lightly cathected processes occur and can still influence the individual's behavior; we call them unconscious.

The amount of object and ego cathexes invested into the impact will determine whether or not the result will be conscious and whether it is minimally or strongly experienced consciously, hence the vividness of our attention to it. If we are tired and our available ego cathexis is low, we can miss much of a conversation, although the conversants may be talking in a sufficiently loud voice. We just won't hear them. The deeply involved sleeper, with almost all the cathexis removed from his ego boundaries, may require the long and loud ringing of an alarm clock to bring him back to a state of consciousness. On the other hand, the hunter who is highly alert (whose ego boundaries are strongly cathected) attends to the slightest sound of a twig moved by a hidden deer. And the highly cathected "third ear" (Reik, 1948) of the sensitive analyst picks up the subtle undertones of unconscious communication from the associations of the patient.

In the case of *repression* it may well be that the ego utilizes certain energies to forcefully counteract the sensitivity of its perceiving boundaries, so that it is unable to experience the offending, impacting objects, thoughts, motivations, affects, etc. They then become unconscious.

TRANSITORY VERSUS PERMANENT INTROJECTS

The question might be asked why some relationships with other individuals turn into permanent introjects (object representations), constant entities with a long-lasting influence (like critical parents), while others are transitory, leaving no crystalized internal structure that continues to contact and influence the self. Perhaps this might be related to the strength of the impact. The effect on us of a very significant individual may so alter the structure of the ego as to leave a permanent residual in the same way that the touch of a very hot iron on the skin leaves a burn and permanent scar tissue.

When the impact of an external object on the perceptual ego boundary is comparatively light (like the influence of a less-than-important person or one with whom our relationship is brief), an introject if formed may be transitory. Like the touch of a lukewarm object, though sensed, it leaves no permanent effect. The issue here is economic, one related to the magnitude of the impact, hence, the quantity of cathexes involved, both subject and object.

THE DIRECTIONALITY OF ENERGIES

Federn also characterized cathexes by their directionality as well as whether they possessed the sense of selfness (ego cathexis) or lacked that selfness (object cathexis). He employed the terms *libido* and *mortido*. By libido Federn meant an integrating, building (loving) force that brought elements together and constructed higher-order levels of organic complexity. This was not the same as Freud's use of the term (1923) to represent a sexual energy, even though sex implies a togetherness of two individuals.

Mortido, on the other hand, represented a dividing, repelling (destroying) force that tended to separate entities and reduce organisms back to their simple origins (death). These two directionalities in cathectic energies might be compared to centripetal (drawing together) gravitational movements versus centrifugal (flinging apart) movements in heavenly bodies, or to the attraction of plus to minus magnetic fields as opposed to the repelling of minus to minus magnetic fields.

The investing of images with mortidinal object cathexes at low levels permits their differentiation from each other by the perceiver and could be regarded as constructive, for example, the ability to distinguish between the perception of another individual and the introject of that person.

The innervating of different ideas by libidinal ego cathexis would permit their cognitive integration, since they would tend to be drawn together. The clustering of different behavioral and experiential items within an ego state occurs because of their common ego cathecting. Complete common cathecting of all such elements might result in such a thorough integration or fusion as to prevent an individual from distinguishing between his right and left hand. Thus, as in most psychological processes (like anxiety), which at lower levels are adaptive, excess tends to make for maladaptiveness.

"SELF" ENERGIES

According to Federn, the *core of the ego* is invested primarily with ego cathexis. Its boundaries consist of object cathexes or mortidinal ego cathexes, which, by their repelling nature, keep the self within and the non-self outside. If this were not so, there could be no boundaries and the self energies would simply flow back into the universe, undifferentiated and without identity. The individual person would cease to exist as such.[4] J. Watkins (1978a) has pursued this line of thought further, but we will not do so again here because its implications do not appear to be significantly relevant to the practice of ego state therapy described here.

Suffice it to summarize at this point that Federn posited two kinds or qualities of cathexes, an ego or self (organic) energy and an object, non-self (inorganic) energy. Either of these cathexes may have a libidinal (attracting, togetherness) directionality or a mortidinal (separating, repelling) tendency.

Federn suggested further that ego cathexis could be *active*, as in planning, thinking, and doing, or *passive*, as determining the need to receive stimuli. He also spoke of *reflexive* ego cathexis in regard to self-love (libidinal) or self-hate (mortidinal) and of *objectless* or *medial* cathexis as represented in such activities as "I live" or "I develop" (libidinal) or "I age" and "I die" (mortidinal). He affirmed that medial cathexis was the manifestation of primary narcissism, that with which we are born, and that it constitutes the "pleasantly familiar" feeling by which we sense our own existence.

These refinements, elaborations, and extended speculations from his fundamental contribution, the concept of dual energies, will not be given much further attention in this book since they do not appear to be relevant to the present status of ego state theory and therapy. It should be noted, however, that investment of any physical or psychological element in an individual may involve partial amounts of either or both ego and object cathexes. When a part of the body, such as a limb, is invested with more object than ego cathexis it will feel strange, as if it were not part of "the me." We experience this during hysterical numbness or paralysis. If conscious, psychological self elements are lacking adequate ego cathexis, we will experience *depersonalization*, which in its extreme form results in the terror felt by psychotics at losing their "self."

HYPNOSIS AND ENERGIES

Within the two-energy theory it is helpful for the therapist to think of hypnosis as a modality for the moving and changing of energies. When one hypnotically suggests to a patient that he is now able to move a hysterically paralyzed limb, this may happen because ego cathexis has now invested it, changing it from object to subject, hence bringing it within the self and voluntary control by the individual.

Likewise, by hypnotically directing more object cathexis into a repressed memory, it becomes strong enough to impact the ego boundary sufficiently as to render it conscious. Cathexes are also moved into an object or process whenever we pay attention to it.

Although Federn himself did not employ hypnosis in his treatment, he foreshadowed its use in ego state therapy. Edoardo Weiss, in his introduction to Federn's book (see Federn, 1952, p. 15), wrote, "Ego states of earlier ages do not disappear, but are only repressed. In hypnosis, a former ego state containing the corresponding emotional dispositions, memories and urges can be re-awakened in the individual."

If a hypnotized subject's hand is made to wag up and down without conscious control, we have simply removed its ego cathexis. It is anesthetic and apparently not within the control of the amused subject. Its movement is now energized by object cathexis. The wagging can become voluntary only if it is ego cathected. Hypnosis thus becomes a powerful therapeutic modality for altering ego and object energy changes within our patients.

PSYCHOSES AND EGO CATHEXES

Perhaps Federn's most significant contribution stemming from his two-energy theory was in the understanding of psychotic symptoms and the psychotherapeutic treatment of psychoses (see Federn, 1952, chapters 6, 7, 8, 9, 10, 11, & 12).

A hallucination is a pseudoperception. The schizophrenic actually sees, hears, or otherwise senses something that does not really exist in the outer world. To the mentally ill patient these perceptions appear to be quite real, as can be well verified by the clinician who tries to persuade him otherwise. Yet the stimuli from which these pseudoperceptions arise come from within the patient, from his own inner cognitions. They represent ideas that are normally experienced as subject, that is, as stemming from one's self. The psychotic, however, experiences them as object and similar to other outside objects that he sees, hears, or otherwise senses.

How can thoughts be turned into perceptions? Federn believed that psychotic patients sense the contents of their delusions and hallucinations as real because they originate from repressed mental stimuli that entered consciousness without obtaining ego cathexis, not because of faulty reality testing. He reasoned that the mental content (idea) was strong enough, hence sufficiently energized, to become conscious, but its original ego energy had been replaced with object cathexis. Accordingly, when it contacted an ego boundary (even though from the inside) it was sensed as an alien element, an object, as the perception of an external object, not as "my" thought.

The problem lay in the weakness of the ego boundary. Like a geographical boundary (e.g., such as between Canada and the United States) that is inadequately manned with border guards, citizens can be mistaken for aliens and vice versa. In the psychotic, the inability to test reality adequately results from an energy deficiency, a lack of sufficient ego cathexis to man the ego boundaries, where the differentiation must be made.

We should help the patient to build more ego energy. He will then be able to remedy this deficiency. That, of course, is precisely what we do with relationship, supportive therapy, exercise, etc. In the implementation of such an approach, Federn often used a nurse, a mother-surrogate, who could provide the nurturing relationship normally received from one's mother (Schwing, 1954).

The importance of the mother figure and her nurturing in developing self-identity and stable object representations, which Federn and Schwing had been emphasizing, has currently begun to receive more attention. Through the concepts of the object-relations theorists, such as Kernberg (1976), Mahler (1975), and Winnicott (1965), who were apparently not aware of Federn's earlier contributions, the significance of mothers as "transitional objects" in the development of self structures in infants is now being increasingly recognized. Baker (1981), Copeland (1986), and Murray-Jobsis (1984) have employed some of these same concepts in treating psychotics within the hypnotic modality.

Federn, and especially his disciple Weiss (1960), stressed the distinction between *reality testing* and the *sensing of reality*. We "sense" reality as something outside our self whenever an object-cathected item impacts an ego boundary. However, to "test" reality we need to move our eyes, ears, and body about and note that the sensed object moves its relative position accordingly. The schizophrenic fails to take this action, relying instead entirely on his weakened ego boundaries to distinguish real from unreal, thoughts from perceptions.

Federn reported that there is a felt difference between the impact of an object on the "inside" of the ego's boundary and its "outside," that which fronts on the external world. This is also true if there is a change in the magnitude of the impact. The psychotic is able to experience this "reality" of his reported experience when it is explained that there are two kinds of reality, "reality A" and "reality B." This approach enlists his cooperation rather than his antagonism at being accused of "lying."

Federn would say to the patient, "When you see me here across the desk I want you to label that 'reality A.' When you see or hear those people who are persecuting you, I want you to call that 'reality B.' Reality A is a kind of experience you can share with others because they, too, are aware of reality A. However, reality B is a private reality which they cannot share. If you talk to them about reality B they will think you are crazy. So when you describe to me any experience, tell me whether it is reality A or reality B."

Federn claimed that psychotic patients could distinguish between reality A and reality B, even though both were experienced as real. By teaching them to make this discrimination he was exercising, strengthening, and hence recathecting their ego boundaries. In time they not only made this distinction, but by not reinforcing reality B, decathected it and returned it to the world of nocturnal dreams, wherein lie the inactive "hallucinations" of normal people. By reducing the energy in reality B, its impact with self boundaries became lower than the threshold necessary to become conscious.

To Federn, psychotic symptoms were a consequence of the necessity to economize one's deficiency of ego cathexis. Psychoanalysis as a treatment modality is contraindicated for psychotics, who are already ego cathexis anemic, since it requires additional energies to uncover and integrate repressed material. In the borderline psychotic, an uncovering, analytic therapy may well precipitate a full-blown psychosis—as has often been verified. This danger can be lessened, however, if the treating one, through a close, intensive "therapeutic self" relationship involving mutual "resonance" (Watkins, 1978a), gives to the patient a "loan" of ego cathexis. The total energy available then may be adequate for him to tolerate the confrontation with his primitive, unegotized material and reintegrate (egotize) it into self structure.

THE ECONOMICS OF SELF[5]

Let us, at least for the moment, accept the concept that self is not a content but simply an energy, which is characterized only by the feeling of "me-ness." Perhaps then what we know about the functioning of other energies (electricity, heat, light, etc.) may suggest ways to better understand self processes and interactions.

An electrical engineer must consider not only the direction and displacements of electricity (as its flow activates lights, motors, and other appliances), but also the quantum required for their proper or full energizing. If there is inadequate electricity flowing into a motor it may not be sufficient to turn it over, or if it does so, it may be sluggish with little zip. During sleep, ego cathexis is apparently at a low ebb; accordingly, there is little self action or experience, perhaps just enough for some internal images in the form of dream activity. If there is a deficiency when we are awake, we may feel sleepy, be less alert than normal, or act schizoid in our behavior.[6] This is similar to a brown-out, which occurs when electricity generation in a region is inadequate to service all the demands of businesses and homes located there. Perhaps this is why the specialist often achieves more in his focused activity than the jack-of-all-trades, whose self energies are spread over a multitude of interests and projects.

We cannot simultaneously be an expert in painting, music, law, psychology, history, politics, business, etc., even though a few individuals in the past, when life was less complex (such as Renaissance man, Leonardo Da Vinci) were able to approach that goal.

Creative people, who can mobilize unusual quantities of ego energies for the activation of their projects, are often considered geniuses. But for all of us the economic factor is ever present. However richly we are endowed with energy, there is a limit, and when we attempt too many activities, or secure inadequate sleep, the quality of our accomplishment suffers.[7]

It may well be that the emptiness (Cushman, 1990) that so many individuals report (sometimes called "existential neurosis") occurs because of the extreme complexity of present-day life. Today, through careers, TV, advertising, reading, organizations, sports, etc., we are all confronted with tremendous demands on our attention. This overstimulation results in inadequate amounts of self energy available for bringing them all vividly into "the me." Cathexis expenditures exceed income, the self becomes anemic, and we are left with a feeling of emptiness. It should be obvious that for any one of us there is an optimum number of interests that should claim our attention and an optimum level of ego investment for maximal functioning.

The question as to where ego and object energies originate is a difficult one. Weiss (1960) believed that both cathexes were generated by metabolic processes, and that the amount which became available resulted from a bifurcation in the metabolism that determined the quantity of each so produced.

At any rate, in planning therapeutic interventions we must consider available cathexes (the economics of self) as well as the psychodynamics of energy disposition.[8] This consideration is especially true as we undertake to treat multiple personality or other dissociations.

Self Derivatives

One addition to Federn's self theory seems indicated. If self is simply an energy, then it has no content or boundaries. Federn (1952) defined pure self (ego feeling) as "the residual experience which persists after the subtraction of all ideational contents." However, when we describe our "selves" we generally attach the word "my" to some specific content with boundaries, for example, "my hand," "my thought," "my beliefs," etc. Accordingly, a term is needed to label mental and physiological entities *after* they have been cathected with self energy. We prefer to call these "self derivatives."

Pure self energy might be viewed as analogous to substance. Substance without modification has no content or boundaries. Ego cathexis has two attributes: As an energy it is capable of activating a process and, as a self energy, that which it cathects is imbued with the feeling of selfness (me-ness). To acquire content and boundaries, this "substance" must be invested into (cathect) some mental or physiological element that does have content and boundaries. Then it takes on the content and boundaries of that cathected element.

A good analogy might be that of paint. Paint has the attribute of adding its color to that which is painted—even as ego cathexis has the attribute of adding the "feeling of selfness" to that which is invested with it. Once colored with a blue paint we then describe the painted chair, wall, or house as a "blue chair," a "blue wall," or a "blue house." Once cathected with self energy, we now have a "self derivative" and can speak of it as "my hand," "my thought," or "my belief."

However, paint only adheres to and colors the external surface of the painted object. Ego cathexis generally infuses the entire physical or psychological entity, perhaps more like something which is drenched with a liquid dye, such that all parts of the entity are imbued with this feeling of selfness. The core self then remains as a storehouse of self energy to be invested into ego states or held in reserve (as during sleep).

3

THE NATURE AND
FUNCTIONING OF EGO STATES

The Discovery of Ego States

Many early contributors had discovered that the human personality is not a unity (although it is usually experienced as such), but is separated into various segments, unique entities that serve different purposes. Janet (1907) applied the term *dissociation* to describe systems of ideas that were split off, thus "not in association" with other ideas within the personality.

Janet had studied true multiple personalities, but he clearly implied that these personality patterns also existed subconsciously, even if not overt and available to conscious observation and experience. Janet, therefore, seems to have been the first to describe those covert personality segments with which we will be primarily concerned in ego state theory and therapy.

A somewhat different but similar approach was formulated by Jung (1969). He described a *complex* as a group of unconscious ideas clustered together. He also described certain, more permanent covert structures within the "collective" or "racial unconscious" that he called *archetypes*. In both terms he implied personality segments that were organized into unconscious patterns.

Federn (1952) was apparently the first contributor to systematically apply the concept of *ego states* in the psychodynamic understanding of behavior. His disciple, Edoardo Weiss (1960), translated his papers, published them, and extended many of their implications. Neither Federn nor Weiss, however, fully realized the great significance of ego states in their treatment procedures.

An ego state may be defined as an organized system of behavior and experience whose elements are bound together by some common principle, and which is separated from other such states by a boundary that is more or less permeable.

Federn included within an ego state only ego-cathected items. However, we have defined it to include both ego-cathected and object-cathected elements, providing they have been organized together into a coherent pattern. This pattern may represent an age or relationship in the individual's life. Or it may have been developed to cope with a certain situation, hence encompassed within a common principle. The ego state must be a collection of subject and object items that belong together in some way and which are included within a common boundary that is more or less permeable.

When one of these states is invested with a substantial quantity of ego cathexis it becomes "the self in the here and now." We say that it is *executive*, and it experiences the other states (if it is aware of them at all) as "he," "she," or "it," since they are then primarily invested with object cathexis. As ego and object cathexes flow from one state to another the behaviors and experiences of the individual change, and we may assign the diagnosis of "multiple personality." Defined in this way, ego states subsume what we call "multiple personalities" but also include other such clusters of mental functioning, which may or may not reach consciousness and directly change behavior.

Ego states may be organized in different dimensions. They may be large and include all the various behaviors and experiences activated in one's occupation. They may be small and include only the behaviors and feelings elicited when attending a baseball game. They may represent current modes of behavior and experience or, as in the case of hypnotic regression, include many memories, postures, feelings, etc., that were apparent only at an earlier age.

Figure 1 represents one possible way of conceptualizing ego states. The center (labeled at the side as No. 1) is rather amorphously defined. It might be considered as the *core ego*, which contains a number of behavioral and experiential items that are more or less constant in the normal individual, and which present to the individual and to the world a fairly consistent determination of the way he and others perceive his "self."

However, the boundaries of this core ego are not rigid but can be expanded or contracted to include more or less psychological material. During active periods the core ego is expanded, extending ego cathexis over more mental structures and processes. The individual then feels and appears to others as vigorous. During rest, sleep, or depression the core ego contracts its boundaries and withdraws ego energies, leaving small or large amounts of behavioral and experiential material external to it, unenergized and dormant. If some of this material is then invested with object cathexis it may be experienced by the individual, but as not-me, like in dreams.

The other ego states depicted in figure 1, with more specifically defined boundaries, may be considered as segments of self that were differentiated for adaptive purposes in the course of normal development. Some may also represent introjects of significant others, or may have been split off from the core ego because of trauma. When the boundaries of such an ego state are

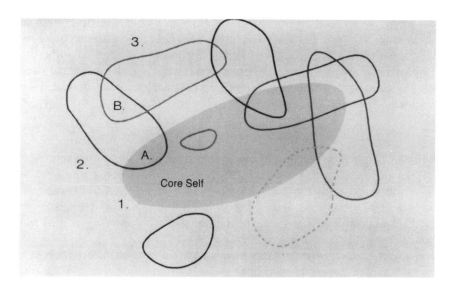

Figure 1. Ego states.

relatively permeable and not rigid, we think of it as a normally adaptive entity. When the boundaries become rigid and impermeable we term it as *dissociated*, which in its extreme form may become the alter of a multiple personality.

Some ego states may be relatively isolated, while others may overlap in content. Note ego states 2 and 3 in figure 1, which overlap on area B. Perhaps ego state 2 was composed of the behaviors and experiences active when the individual was age six, and ego state 3 represents behaviors and experiences dealing with authority figures, including father. Area B would then include those psychological structures and processes that were active when, at age six, he was interacting with his father.

During therapy (by techniques which will be described later) we can activate and move to ego state 3 if we first regress the patient to the age of six (ego state 2) and then focus on experiences with father at that age (area B). For consideration and treatment purposes we can then tap into the individual's interactions with authority figures throughout his life and activate the significant associations.

Some items may be within the boundaries of several ego states. For example, different ego states may use the same English language, but at times with differences in the particular words and accents employed.

Certain words used by adult states may not be within the vocabularies of child states, etc. And behaviors to accomplish a similar goal may be uniquely different from one ego state to another. For example, individuals who are bilingual may speak one language when a certain ego state is executive. When they speak the other language, another ego state may take its place (see chapter 7).

Integration and Differentiation

Human personality develops through two basic processes, integration and differentiation. By *integration* a child learns to put concepts together, such as cow and horse, and thus to build more complex units called animals. By *differentiation* he separates general concepts into more specific meanings, such as discriminating between a cat and a rabbit. Both processes are normal and adaptive.

Normal differentiation permits us to experience one set of behaviors at a party Saturday night and another at the office during the week. When this separating or differentiating process becomes excessive and maladaptive we call it dissociation.

When we differentiate two items, both of which are consciously in mind, we compare them and note their differences. In dissociation the two items are so separated from one another that comparison is not possible, since only one is within consciousness at any given time. Both differentiation and dissociation involve the psychological separating of two entities, but differentiation is lesser in degree, generally adaptive, and considered to be normal. Dissociation, on the other hand, is considered to be pathological. It may be more immediately adaptive but often at the expense of greater maladaptiveness later. These two may be considered as simply resulting from different degrees of "the separating process."

Characteristics of Ego States

To understand and deal with ego states one must consider their origin. Often they were first created when the individual was quite young. Accordingly, they think concretely like a child. Adult logic may not reach them, even though they often talk in an adult voice. It is as if they were frozen in time. Covert ego states, unlike the alters in a true multiple personality, require hypnosis for their activation. But if they first originated when the patient was a child, then one should think of them like a small girl who is dressed up in mother's clothes and pretending to be an adult.

Most adults have lost the ability to think concretely like a child, and thus we are at a disadvantage in dealing with child ego states, especially when they are not so clearly differentiated as true multiple personality alters. States that were created during the subject's adolescence will think like a teenager, rejecting and suspicious of grown-ups and very defensive of their own independence; they don't want to be told what is right or what they ought to do. This characteristic will be more clearly illustrated in case excerpts in later chapters. In dealing with child and adolescent states, one should conceptualize to whom one is talking and conduct the interaction accordingly. The clinician who resonates well (Watkins, J., 1978a) will be more successful.

One should be mindful that a child ego state was formed to adapt to the conditions of yesteryear, not today, and that often its attempts to function today result in maladaptation. As one inquires and secures some information about the time and circumstances when an ego state first appeared, one's approach can be modified accordingly, even though one is confronted ostensibly with a full-grown adult. This modification can be done without embarrassment under hypnosis.

Another characteristic of an ego state is that it was probably developed to enhance the individual's ability to adapt and cope with a *specific* problem or situation. Thus, one ego state may have taken over the overt, executive position when dealing with parents, another on the playground, another during athletic contests, etc.

In the case of a true multiple personality, the specific situation is usually some very severe trauma such as child abuse. An ego state formed to help in dissociating the pain from the primary alter or to make it easier for the major personality to deal with an abuser without inviting retaliation. It is to be expected that these specific ego states will be reactivated in the transferences of the present, such as to teachers, employers, supervisors, colleagues—and therapists (Watkins & Watkins, 1990a).

Another common trait is that once created, ego states are highly motivated to protect and continue their existence. The clinician who tries to eliminate a maladaptive state will find to his dismay that the entity probably does not disappear, but that one's intervention has now created an internal enemy who resists therapeutic intervention. Part-persons seek to protect their existence, as do whole-persons. This tendency has important implications in the treatment of multiple personalities, which will be discussed later. It is much easier to modify the motivations of ego states and change their behavior constructively than it is to attempt their total elimination.

A related corollary to this persistence in existence is to realize that the original ego state came into being to protect and facilitate the adaptation of the primary person. It remained because it had a certain amount of success. And from what we have learned about behavior modification we can recognize that it was positively reinforced, first for coming into existence, then for continuing its being. Never mind that now its efforts may be counterproductive. The earlier conditionings will hold precedence.

We must recognize the differences in the environment of the past and that of today. One cannot generally induce a state to change into an adaptive stance toward today's adult problems when its earlier struggles are not understood by the treating clinician. Recognition of these traits are essential in the planning and conduct of effective therapeutic maneuvers (such as abreactions).

Often when working with ego states the internal equilibrium of the subject will change in such a way that a new ego state (or one which has been long dormant) will be energized and will make itself known. This state may first manifest itself by slight changes in posture, mannerism, or voice pitch.

Returning to the two-energy theory of Federn, the nature of the problems of the past determined the creation and cathexis of the various states. The adaptational needs of the present must be met with the appropriate dispositions of object and ego energies assisted by an understanding therapist. Hypnosis is a modality that facilitates this allocation of subject and object energies. The effective accomplishment of this treatment goal, utilizing the many tactics of supportive, behavioral, psychoanalytic, cognitive, and existential therapies, constitutes the approach we have called ego state therapy.

Ego states that are cognitively dissonant from one another or have contradictory goals frequently develop conflicts with each other. When they are highly energized and have rigid, impermeable boundaries, multiple personalities may result. However, many such conflicts appear between ego states only covertly, and are frequently manifested by anxiety, depression, or any number of neurotic symptoms and maladaptive behaviors.

The Development of Ego States

Ego states apparently develop by one or more of the following three processes: normal differentiation, introjection of significant others, and reactions to trauma.

First, through *normal differentiation* the child learns to discriminate foods that taste good and those that do not. He not only makes these simple discriminations, but many others as well, and develops entire patterns of behavior that are appropriate for dealing with parents, teachers, and playmates, and adaptive for adjusting to school, the playground, etc.

These changes are considered quite normal, yet they do represent syndromes of behavior and experience that are clustered and organized under some common principle. As such, they can be considered ego states. The boundaries between these entities and other personality patterns are very flexible and permeable. The child in school is quite aware (or easily capable of becoming aware) of himself in a playground situation. Playground behaviors, however, are not as easily activated when at the school desk (in the presence of the teacher). There is resistance at the boundaries. These less-clearly differentiated ego states are usually adaptive and are economic in providing appropriate behavior patterns when needed.

Second, through the *introjection of significant others* the child erects clusters of behavior, which if ego-cathected become roles that he himself experiences, and if object-cathected represent inner objects with whom he must relate and interact. For example, if he introjects a punishing parent and hence develops an ego state pattern around his perceptions of that parent, he may be constantly depressed as he tries to cope covertly with an inward continuation of the accusations and abuse originally heaped upon him by the real parent. However, if later he ego-cathects this state (e.g., infuses it with self-energy) he will not suffer, but he will abuse his own children. We would then say he has "identified" with his bad parent.

He not only introjects the abusing parent, but he may also introject the drama of the original parent-child conflict. Whether he suffers from this internalization or identifies with it and inflicts suffering on others will depend on whether it is primarily object-cathected or ego-cathected. An individual with multiple personalities may alternate between these two patterns of response. Finally, if he introjects both his mother and father, and if these two parents were constantly quarreling with each other, then he may internalize their conflict. This might be manifested by constant headaches of whose origin he is unaware as the two parental ego states battle with each other.

Third, when confronted with severe *trauma*, rejection, or abuse, the child may dissociate. A lonesome youngster often removes the ego cathexis from part of himself, reenergizes it with object cathexis, and creates an imaginary playmate with whom he can interact. Most children with imaginary playmates discard or repress these entities upon going to school. But if such an ego state is merely repressed, later conflict and environmental pressure may cause it to be reinvested with energy and to reemerge, perhaps in a malevolent, self-punishing form, as it did in the case of Rhonda Johnson, who coauthored with me (JGW) her life story and treatment in *We, the Divided Self* (Watkins & Johnson, 1982).

The Differentiation-Dissociation Continuum

Few psychological processes exist on an either-or basis. Anxiety, depression, immaturity, etc., all lie on a continuum with lesser or greater degrees of intensity. So it is with differentiation-dissociation. Multiple personality only represents the extreme and maladaptive end of the continuum that starts with normal differentiation.

Figure 2 illustrates this continuum. Toward the left, the three ego states (A, B, C) are separated by a very permeable boundary. This is the situation we find in most normal people. The different states share much content in common and are quite aware of each other. They are experienced as common mood changes. As we move to the right on this continuum the boundaries separating the states become more rigid. It is probable that the best personality adjustment occurs a little to the right from the extreme left (where there would be no boundaries, and thus no separate ego states). Differentiation is adaptive, and some separation of personality segments should make for better personality functioning. Otherwise, it would be like an office in which all papers are thrown together and not separated into classified files.

On the extreme right the boundaries become so impermeable that the ego state segments have little or no interaction, communication, or shared content. When one is executive it is unaware of the existence of the others. Each, when activated, becomes a true multiple personality alter.

In the condition just to the left of this true MPD (DID) we have a borderline multiple. The various states are conscious of the existence of each other but refer to the others as "he," "she," or "it," and not as "me." This position on the differentiation-dissociation continuum represents a bordering (almost true) multiple personality, and is not to be confused with the diagnosis of borderline personality.

EGO STATES

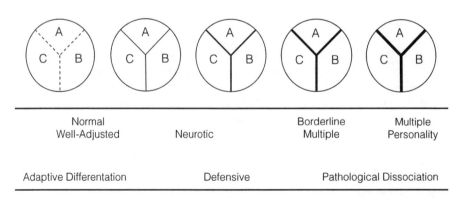

Figure 2. The differentiation-dissociation continuum.

In between are ego states which, because of lesser degrees of rigidity in the semipermeable boundaries, retain partial communication, interaction, and sharing of content. In general, they remain covert and do not spontaneously appear overtly, but they can be activated into the executive position by hypnosis.

In this region we find that a conflict between states may be manifested by headaches, anxiety, and maladaptive behaviors, such as found in the neuroses and psychophysiologic conditions. It is in this area where the most productive contributions of ego state concepts to psychotherapy have occurred. We are therefore concerned with a general principle of personality formation in which the dispositions of the activating energies and the impermeability of the boundaries separating the organized ego-state patterns have resulted in relatively discrete personality segments that may alternate in assuming the executive position, experienced as "the self" in "the now." The extreme form of this separating process results in true multiple personalities (now called dissociative identity disorder) in the *DSM-IV* [APA, 1994].

Multiple personalities have traditionally been considered to be extremely rare. However, many reports of cases are now being presented that, although the disorder may be uncommon, it can no longer be considered rare (APA, 1994).

Ego States and Multiple Personalities

It is important for the therapist who is working with either multiple personalities or covert ego-state conflicts not to create artifacts through suggestion. Although ego states will often give themselves names, as do true multiple personalities, we are careful not to suggest names but let them emerge as nondirectively as possible.

Too many practitioners today are hypnotically activating covert ego states and announcing that they have discovered another multiple personality. We have often found covert ego states among normal students who volunteer for hypnotic studies. Even though multiple personalities are usually studied through hypnosis, they should be so diagnosed only when the ego states can become overt spontaneously, without the use of hypnosis. We also consider it essential that there be evidence of amnesia in the present. For example a patient with MPD may say that he was reported to have been at a ballgame yesterday but can't recall being there. In fact, he may be quite adamant that everyone else must be mistaken, yet cannot ascertain himself where he was that afternoon. Such lapses of time will be evident in the history of a patient with true MPD.

These consistencies of behavior within a single state and differences between different states are most clearly observed in true multiple personalities. The Ken personality in the "Hillside Strangler" (Watkins, J., 1984) always smoked filtertip cigarettes and held them between the first and second fingers, palm toward the face. The Steve personality always tore the filters off and held the cigarette between the thumb and first finger, palm away from the face. Bianchi continued to show this same alternation of behavior during the first years of his subsequent incarceration in prison when he had nothing to gain by claiming a psychiatric defense.

The relationship between multiple personalities and ego states as found in normal individuals was demonstrated to us through posttherapy reactions given by successfully treated multiples. In these cases, presumably integrated, separate dissociated entities no longer appeared spontaneously. A former patient, when asked about one of her other personalities, simply said, "She was me." The reaction was much like what one would say if asked about one's behavior at a party last week. The previous dissociating boundaries were now sufficiently permeable so that the patient could experience her earlier behaviors as part of her self. Ego cathexis could now move easily from one state to the other.

However, this did not mean that there had been a "fusion," wherein no boundaries existed at all. This point was well brought out by another multiple patient at the conclusion of treatment. When she was again hypnotized, the previous entities reappeared but stated, "We aren't separate persons any more. We are just parts of her." In other words, the former multiple had the same segments, but they were now separated by very permeable boundaries, just as they are in normal volunteer research subjects. The personality segments had become normal ego states, accessible only under hypnosis, and the individual had simply moved along the differentiation-dissociation continuum from maladaptive dissociation toward adaptive differentiation.

This suggests that perhaps the most efficient treatment of multiple personalities does not come by aiming at a complete fusion, since normal people manifest ego states that are differentiated and not fused. To seek only fusion in treatment would be like trying to induce the Arabs and the Israelis to unite in one single, big nation, rather than to communicate, cooperate, and coexist peacefully. It is not surprising that when this tactic has been attempted in the past with multiple personalities, their forced integration was unstable and they soon dissociated again. We had this experience with earlier cases.

A more economic approach is to move our patient back along the differentiation-dissociation continuum (see figure 2) by reducing rigidity of the state boundaries, lessening the conflicts between ego states, and promoting mutual understanding through interstate communication, much as we would do in family therapy. We do not then have to struggle with the resistance that the various ego states maintain to protect their individual identity and existence, a separateness originally created by attempts at adaptive differentiation. We recognize the original needs but turn them in constructive directions. Our therapeutic task becomes much easier since ego states, like whole people, fight very hard to retain their identities. As "Steve" in the Bianchi case said to me (JGW), "I don't like you. You're trying to get rid of me." Only after I assured him otherwise did I get the confidence and cooperation that resulted in his (Steve's) confession to the many murders in Los Angeles (Watkins, J., 1984).

By not challenging their unique identity, but by increasing the communication of ego states with each other, we encourage an adaptive togetherness. The formerly dissociated multiple personality becomes a normal individual differentiated into cognitively consonant ego states which cooperate in adjusting to the individual's inner and outer worlds. Often though, many of the original alters, when their need for separateness no longer exists, will disappear spontaneously, their contents fusing into remaining ones. The remaining differentiated entities are now simply covert ego states—and the individual consistently manifests only one "personality" overtly.

Ego states that are cognitively dissonant from one another or have contradictory goals often develop conflicts with each other. When they are highly energized and have rigid, impermeable boundaries, multiple personalities may develop. Many such conflicts appear between ego states that are only covert. These may be manifested by anxiety, depression, or any number of neurotic symptoms and maladaptive behaviors. Overeating and obesity often result from pressures on the main, executive personality by a disgruntled, covert ego state. These conflicts require a kind of internal diplomacy not unlike what we do in treating true multiple personalities. However, since the contending ego states do not spontaneously appear overtly, they must generally be activated through hypnosis. We call this ego state therapy.

Ego state therapy is the utilization of individual, family, and group therapy techniques for the resolution of conflicts between the different ego states that constitute a "family of self" within a single individual. It is a kind of internal diplomacy that may employ any of the directive, behavioral, cognitive, analytic, or humanistic techniques of treatment, usually under hypnosis.

Hypnosis and Ego States

Hypnosis is both a focusing and dissociative process (Hilgard, 1986). Through hypnosis we can focus on one segment of personality and temporarily ablate or dissociate away other parts. In fact, since hypnosis itself is a form of dissociation, it is not surprising to find that good hypnotic subjects often manifest covert ego-state segments in their personalities, and they are not mentally ill. Hypnosis offers access to levels of personality which in classical psychoanalysis require much longer periods of time to contact.

Since ego state therapy is an approach involving interpart communication and diplomacy, hypnosis becomes almost a sine qua non for practicing it when the states are covert.

Ego States and Hidden Observers

Hilgard (1977) discovered that a hypnotic subject in which deafness had been suggested, when told to lift a finger if he could still hear at some level, did so. He also found that when pain was presumably eliminated by hypnotic analgesia, the subject, through finger signals, reported that he could (unconsciously) still perceive the discomfort.

Hilgard held that this represented a covert, cognitive structural system, and he called it *the hidden observer*. We have found that when Hilgard's hidden observers have been activated in normal college students who volunteered as hypnotic subjects, further inquiry into their nature and content has usually elicited organized ego states. In one set of experiments, we activated hidden observers in former ego state therapy patients using the same procedures and verbalizations employed by Hilgard in his studies, repeating with both hypnotic deafness and hypnotic analgesia. What emerged were various ego states with which we had dealt in treatment over a year earlier (Watkins & Watkins, 1979–80, 1980). We therefore consider that hidden observers and ego states are the same class of phenomena. In chapter 7, verbatim extracts of an actual case from that study are presented (see Watkins & Watkins, 1979–80, 1980). We have also compared hidden observers, ego states, and multiple personalities in more detail in another publication (Watkins & Watkins, 1992).

To finish this discussion of ego state theory, let us note the differences between Federn's original conception of ego states and our view of them as they function in therapy. To Federn, the ego remained a constant, but different contents could pass into and out of it by being ego-cathected. The movement was by these contents, which were then organized by the ego into ego states. When an ego state was decathected of self-energy it retained its organization and continuous existence as an object representation, and was perceived as such. An ego state consisted only of self-cathected items.

In our conception, the self consists of pure ego energy (ego-cathexis), not contents, such as motivations, affects, ideas, etc. This cathexis is not the energy of the self, it *is* the self. When this ego energy passes into contents, these are then experienced as part of the self, as "me." The movement is on the part of the self-energy as it passes into and out of various organized behavior and experience patterns called ego states. Such a state may contain both object and self representations, which on repression (removed from consciousness) still retain their respective and relative structures. This ego state, whether self- or object-cathected, is the unit to be dealt with in therapy. It takes on the character of the major amount of cathexis within it, ego or object, and is experienced by the individual as such, "me" or "it."

4

DISSOCIATION

As I walked out the gate, I had the same odd sensation that I'd experienced for much of the afternoon: a dissociation from my actions. It was a kind of out-of-body experience, as though I stood watching at a safe remove while Schwarzkopf went back outside the perimeter, at a risk of being blown away. But there was nothing eerie or mystical about it. I was kind of on automatic pilot.

Norman H. Schwarzkopf (1992)

In the 1994 Super Bowl, the Buffalo Bills running back, Thurman Thomas, dropped the ball, which was recovered by a Dallas Cowboy player and carried for a touchdown.

News item, Associated Press, February 3, 1994: "As Thomas said, 'The fumble really turned the game around.' Even as he pronounced the self-indictments, he did it with such a curious detachment that a reporter whispered to a friend, "He's talking like it happened to somebody else." Maybe Thomas and the Bills are dealing with pain by distancing themselves from it.

Dissociation can be a very normal reaction, protecting us from frightening situations and lowering our fear. Although often associated with childhood trauma, it can equally affect adults (Cardeña & Spiegel, 1993). It removes from within ourselves an area of conflict. For example, in out-of-body experiences, a not uncommon form of dissociation, we feel ourselves as watchers, not participants, in a dangerous situation. For the moment, the self becomes only an object. We do not have to suffer externally initiated pain or internal fright.

Dissociation itself has had considerable investigation, both clinically and experimentally. Broad surveys of the field have been published by Hilgard (1986, 1992), Wolman and Ullman (1986), and Michelson and Ray (1996). Goettman, Greaves, and Coons (1994) have compiled a most complete bibliography of studies covering the period of 1791 to 1994. These studies run

38

into the hundreds, so we will review only those contributions that bear most directly on the area and thesis of this book.

Hypnosis has been regarded as a form of dissociation (Hilgard, 1986) and has been widely used in the treatment of many disorders including multiple personality (Brown & Fromm, 1986; Fromm, Erika, 1984; Fromm & Nash, 1997; Fromm & Shor, 1979; Watkins, J., 1987, 1992b). It is also often used in the practice of ego state therapy—which itself is an extension of hypnoanalysis.

Dissociation is a separating process that extends throughout a continuum from normal and adaptive differentiation to the other extreme of pathological dissociation, like multiple personality disorder (Braun, 1988a, 1988b). Braun has also pointed out that dissociation can occur in one or more specific spheres, such as "behavior, affect, sensation, and knowledge." He called this the BASK theory of dissociation.

Ego state theory also uses the concept of a continuum of the separating tendency but denotes its various stages of intensity somewhat differently (Watkins, J., 1992a, 1992b), which will be described in later chapters. In ego state therapy we will be more concerned with its intermediate manifestations. However, any process is often best studied when attention is first given to its most severe forms. Accordingly, let us consider the dissociative diagnoses of amnesia and multiple personality.

Amnesia

Amnesia[1] occurs commonly in patients with multiple personalities. However, non-MPD cases, where it is the only or primary symptom, are often quite dramatic, but they occur infrequently. Nevertheless, there are a number of reports of "pure" amnesia cases in the literature (see Akhtar, Lindsey, & Kahn, 1991; Brna & Wilson, 1990; Coons & Milstein, 1992; Christianson & Nilsson 1984; Eisen, 1989; Gill & Rapaport, 1942; and Knowles, 1964).

Unlike multiple personality disorders, amnesia seems to be related to immediate adult adjustment problems rather than the consequences of early child abuse. The patient is confronted with a situation with which he cannot cope. He may solve the dilemma by blocking out the entire present and past, often losing his identity.

A man in the Tacoma, Washington, area was reported in a news item as being picked up in another town living under a different name. The report stated that on being returned to his family, he was unable to recognize his wife and children. Such nonrecognition is a clue to the cause of his amnesia. He apparently sought to eliminate his family, perhaps because he could not adjust to married life.

A case with which one of us (JGW) was more familiar was that of a soldier who blacked out in combat. On "coming-to" he had lost his identity and was hospitalized. After many attempts through drugs and hypnosis to help him regain his memories, he was sent home. He was unable to recognize family and friends, and returned to the hospital. Following an implied threat that if he did not recover his memories he might be sent back into combat (so he could regain his memories where he lost them), he relinquished the amnesia, and his memory returned. (The case is described in more detail in Watkins, J., 1949, 1992b).

A follow-up inquiry was answered by his wife, who described him as being hostile and noncooperative with his family. The point is illustrated in that he was dragged back unwillingly to a family situation which the amnesia was designed to escape. The case illustrates that merely reinstating memory, perhaps by hypnotic suggestion, is poor therapy if it is not followed or accompanied by a reexamination of the unbearable situation from which the patient escaped by amnesia. The symptom is relieved, but not its original cause, a condition which is still present and capable of causing further maladjustment.

Sometimes the patient will be in a situation with which he is having difficulty coping, but amnesia appears only after it has been precipitated by some physical accident. A young man involved with a homosexual gang suffered a motorcycle accident on his way home from the funeral of a gang member who was killed in a motorcycle accident. The patient, on awakening in the hospital and suffering severe head damage, was unable to remember any of his previous life. He also experienced considerable aphasia.

Through hypnotic suggestion under regression, he was able to remember not only the more immediate present, but also his childhood and growing up. However, unlike the first case, relief of the primary symptom was followed by an abreactive reliving of the accident and a hypnoanalytic working-through of the homosexual conflict. This situation was resolved by insight therapy and he made peace with himself. As a result he returned to life with good adjustment and went on to become self-supporting.

This case taught the therapist that even though the symptom followed known brain trauma (he had a plate in his head), and was accompanied by observable brain damage, aphasia, the primary symptom of amnesia was psychologically based. It was developed under cover of a recognized organic impairment that served to conceal the real cause of his amnesia, and which could well have resulted in no attempt at psychotherapy.

PRINCIPLES IN THE TREATMENT OF AMNESIA

After hypnotic induction and considerable deepening, the patient should be regressed to an early age, one far preceding the onset of the amnesia. Work slowly up the age ranges with recollection of a number of incidents at different ages. Use the present tense to get the patient into each scene ("What's he saying to you?"). Talk at the level and with the vocabulary that you expect the patient would have used at the regressed age. Break down the amnesic barrier by poking holes in it at various ages ("You're in the third grade. You can see the teacher in front of you. What's her name?").

First try recall: "What's happening?" If the patient does not respond or says, "I don't know," move to recognition: "What does the person look like?" Try a projective technique: "Something's happening. What's coming to mind?" or "Whom do you like best?" If an accident was the precipitating incident, establish remembering and reliving just prior to it. When approaching a traumatic event, go slowly in great detail to get the patient fully involved. Suggest the affect at the time of the trauma: "You're right there and it's happening now." Try: "You're thinking out loud." If fear is apparent from nonverbal cues, anticipate the patient's inner feelings and mental state: "You're scared." Involve yourself in the fearful scene: "What are we going to do now?" Build up tension in your own voice appropriate to the situation: "Look out! Look out!" Repeat important sentences: "He's hitting me!" By such repetition the patient hears what he or she has just said, and it promotes movement without suggestion from the therapist.

In the abreacting of traumatic incidents, let the experience and the accompanying feelings run to exhaustion. Ask the patient if she is willing to remember the event post-hypnotically; if there is agreement, bring her out of hypnosis with the suggestion for remembering. After arousal have the patient consciously recall the event with all its details. If she is unwilling, suggest that recall will occur when she is ready to remember.

Review the situation under hypnosis, during the same session if possible. Review it again 24 hours later. Also review it a week later if needed. Note details to see if it is remembered in the same way. Later recall may involve more or less details. Since confabulation of hypnotically secured memories (Loftus, 1993; Watkins, J., 1989, 1993a) is possible, check to see consistency, especially if the lifting of the amnesia is for a court case. Court cases regarding memories hypnotically refreshed have become quite controversial in recent years (Mutter, 1990; Orne, 1984; Pettinati, 1988; Watkins, J., 1993a).[2]

In such forensic cases, record the entire time, preferably with videotape. Amnesia should be regarded as the symptom of an underlying and unresolved life problem. In a therapy case, follow up resolution of the amnesia by investigating and working through the underlying life problems and conflicts with traditional psychotherapy, so that the patient will be prepared to adjust to the situations with which previously he or she could not cope. Otherwise, one risks the possibility that the amnesia or equivalent symptoms will return.

Amnesia is common in multiple personality cases, since the primary personality, not being present when an underlying alter is "out," will have little or no memory of what transpired during that time. However, we will treat that amnesia as part of the dissociated MPD condition and not separately.

Multiple Personality Disorder (Dissociative Identity Disorder)

Multiple personality was once considered a very rare disorder. Before the 1970s very few cases were reported. In the last 20 years there has been a renewed interest. The International Society for the Study of Dissociation (ISSD) has been formed and now has over 3,000 members. Interest in MPD has still been limited in other countries (Frischholz, Braun, Martinez-Taboos, Ross, & Van der Hart, 1990; Takahashi, 1990, Van der Hart, 1990, 1993; Van der Hart & Boon, 1990). The clinical and research reports on MPD have become quite voluminous (see Boor & Coons, 1983; Kluft, 1994; Loewenstein, 1989; Prince, 1905/1929); Putnam, Guroff, Silberman, Barban, & Post, 1986; Ross & Loewenstein, 1992; Schreiber, 1974), and there are a number of excellent textbooks now available (e.g., Bliss, 1986; Braun, 1984, 1986; Kluft & Fine, 1993; Putnam, 1989; and Ross, 1989–this is not an exhaustive list). For a "complete" bibliography of literature on the subject, covering from 1791 to 1992, see Goettman, Greaves, and Coons (1994). Accordingly, we shall not attempt to give a comprehensive survey of the field; rather, our aim in this chapter and the following one is to show what we have learned from the study of MPD (DID)[3] patients and the behavior of their alters that can apply to the ego state therapy of less pathological cases, those found in the intermediate range of the differentiation-dissociation continuum.

ORIGINS OF MULTIPLE PERSONALITY DISORDER

Child abuse, whether physical, sexual, and/or psychological, appears to be the fundamental cause of multiple personality (Sands, 1994) In fact, dissociation itself, whether severe enough to cause a true multiple personality or not, seems to be related to trauma and stress (Anderson, 1992; Coons, Bowman, & Milstein, 1988; Frischholz, 1985; Gross & Ratner, 1989; Sanders, McRoberts, & Tollefson, 1989; Spiegel, D., 1993).

Almost always the therapist of a patient with multiple personalities hears tales of childhood horror (Wilbur, D., 1984), and most authorities in the field, with a few exceptions (see Ganaway, 1995), consider that dissociative identity disorder is rooted in severe child abuse (Kluft, 1984; Ross et al.,

1991). There is frequently an amnesia for such memories in the early stages of treatment.

As treatment progresses, more alters may make their presence known. Usually between 5 and 15 such subpersonalities are discovered. However, some clinicians have reported 50 or more. Because of the strong possibility that a dissociating patient will produce many small personality fragments when the discovery of each new one seems to please the therapist, one should be skeptical of such cases (Kluft, 1988; Putnam, 1992). The major variance is usually contained within a much smaller group to which the therapist's attention should be primarily directed.

The diagnosis of MPD (dissociative identity disorder) becomes an especially controversial task when it involves a defendant who is accused of a crime— which he apparently did while in a dissociated state (Orne, 1984; Savitz, 1990). Judges tend to be very skeptical of the reality of MPD and are concerned that this diagnosis will be used by an individual to claim innocence by reason of mental illness, and thus escape responsibility for wrongdoing. Courts tend to equate this condition with conscious malingering.

While every case is unique in the experiences endured, a typical patient might demonstrate something of the following: In early life, usually prior to school, the child was victimized by an adult, more often a male who sexually abused the little one, perhaps even including actual rape. This may also be accompanied by violence, such as severe beatings, and sometimes outright torture. Frequently the abuser threatens the child with even more dire consequences if she (more commonly a girl) reveals this abuse to the mother or anyone else.

The terrified child has only three options: She can die, and some children do; she can disintegrate into a complete psychosis, and some children do; or she can dissociate, which is the most intelligent and adaptive response.

Dissociation involves splitting off a part of "self," turning it from self or subject into non-self or object. In terms of Federn's two-energy theory this would involve removing ego energies from the abusing experiences and cathecting them with object energy, then repressing them.

Now the little one can enjoy a reasonably normal existence with the remaining personality segment executive. By forgetting and repressing the painful experiences she can play the role of a dutiful child. This role does not threaten the aggressor—and perhaps might appease him into treating her better.

The child has now learned a lesson for survival and a way of dealing with future problems. The technique of dissociation has received a positive reinforcement, and is likely to be employed again in the future, perhaps to meet other problems that are difficult but not as life-threatening. A dissociating way of life has been formed. In time, more alters may appear in response to new unpleasant situations that confront the child. By the time the individual has reached adolescence a number of well-defined alters or subpersonalities have been established. These alters view the main personality and each other as objects. They are frequently given names and may engage in competition to be executive, that is, to be "out" and appear as the personality of the moment.

The Diagnosis of Multiple Personality Disorder

Some clinicians do not recognize multiple personality disorder as a legitimate psychiatric entity, and there has been considerable controversy on this issue (APA, 1988; Bliss, 1984; Coons, 1986; Dawson, 1990; Dell, 1988; Fahy, 1988; Hilgard, 1988; Kluft, 1992).

There have been many psychophysiological studies investigating differences in cerebral blood flow, galvanic skin response, response to medication, perception, visual functioning, visual evoked potentials, and in posture, voice, and motor behavior within MPD alters (Braun, 1983; Miller & Triggiano, 1992; Putnam, 1984). Some of the studies did not find differences. However, others reported consistent differences between the responses of different alters within the same individual. Many of the reports are anecdotal and others are demographic. There are a number of experimental investigations, but many of these have design flaws, and the existence of valid and reliable physiologic indicators is still to be determined. Nevertheless, as more practitioners are finding and recognizing these cases, the psychiatric and psychological professions are coming increasingly to accept the reality of a diagnosis of multiple personality disorder. This diagnosis is now called dissociative identity disorder in the *DSM-IV* (APA, 1994) to reflect current consideration of the altered states as *fragments* of a single personality rather than as *separate personalities* inhabiting the same body (Putnam, 1992). The thought processes, feelings, and behaviors of the respective alters appear to be so very different from one another that it is difficult to conceive of them as merely simulated or malingered.

The effect upon a clinician when he or she is first confronted with an MPD patient is usually one of astonishment. In fact, the patient may have been in treatment with that practitioner for a long time, perhaps several months or more, before underlying alters become overt. Perhaps this delay occurred because these entities, having been split off during early painful and abusive treatment, must develop much trust in the therapist before emerging. It is also the reason why skeptical clinicians seldom report finding MPD cases (Koch, 1985; Sarbin, 1995). There is a constant testing of the realness of the

therapist's sincerity, which continues over and over as the treatment progresses (Finch, 1990; LaCalle, 1991). Furthermore, there will be much difference in the trust evinced by certain alters than by others, those who were
likely created during the periods of most severe abuse. Some alters will trust a
woman therapist, but not a man, and others vice versa.

The clinician's first (and continuous) task will be to establish as trusting a
relationship as possible. This may even mean placing distance between him-
or herself and the patient until the treated individual can tolerate more closeness.

In establishing the diagnosis a number of criteria require consideration.
The reported frequency of amnesia is perhaps the most noticeable of these.
When the patient has sufficient trust in the examiner she will often state that
she never declared these amnesic episodes to previous clinicians or others
because, "They'd have thought I was crazy." This reticence is also why court
cases (Watkins, J., 1976, 1978a, 1984) may never have had a verified record
of dissociation prior to the commission of a crime, a fact used by prosecutors
and their expert witnesses to argue that the individual is lying or simulating
MPD in order to escape punishment (Orne, Dinges, & Orne, 1984).

As indicated in chapter 3, the spontaneous emergence of an alter, without
the use of hypnosis, needs to be in evidence in order to diagnose a true MPD.
Otherwise, we consider it an ego state problem, for which the *DSM-IV* code
of "Dissociative Disorder not Otherwise Specified" would be appropriate.

Individuals suffering from MPD frequently report headaches. These headaches tend to occur just prior to switching from the host personality to an
alter or from one alter to another. In some cases the emerging alter will
describe this as a struggle between two entities, one striving to assume the
overt, executive position, and the other battling to hold on to it.

This situation was quite clearly demonstrated when I first became acquainted with the multiplicity in Kenneth Bianchi, the "Hillside Strangler"
(Watkins, J., 1984).[4]

During my second diagnostic evaluation session with him, Kenneth, the
primary state, reported having headaches and "feeling bad." He had experienced a need to go to the bathroom, and after returning continued as follows:

B: I had explained, Dr. Watkins, the reason I left was that I started to
   feel—I don't know why, I started to feel uncomfortable and nervous
   and, matter of fact, even to the point of a little . . . not angry or
   upset, say "agitated," but something inside of me was just boiling.
   I'm sorry I just ran out like that.
W: That's okay, I understand; do you feel okay now?
B: Yes. I do.

After my first session with Bianchi some evaluators felt I had hypnotically suggested an MPD alter (Steve) and had, therefore, created an artifact. Accordingly, this time I was determined to see if the alter Steve would emerge spontaneously with no naming or direct suggestion on my part, and when Bianchi was not under hypnosis. His strange reaction suggested another internal conflict for control, like his repeated headaches. Accordingly, I asked him simply to close his eyes and "feel comfortable."

> W: I was sort of wondering why that feeling of uncomfortableness, and perhaps, uh, uh, I could know more why that uncomfortableness is there?

Bianchi paused some time, then slowly lowered his head. After another minute he suddenly jerked his head up again with a startled look.

> W: Yes?
> B: Yes, what? Hi.
> W: Hi. Are you Ken?
> B: [With an angry, hostile look] Do I look like Ken?
> W: Well, no. Do you know who I am?
> B: Sure. I know who you are.
> W: Okay. You look like you're a little bit disturbed to me.
> B: So what?
> W: We just want to understand each other.
> B: I don't like you. I don't like you at all.
> W: Why don't you like me, Ken? It isn't Ken is it?
> B: No, it's not! It's Steve.

The interview continued with an individual who was totally different in manner, posture, speech, phrases, accent, etc. than the Ken Bianchi with whom I had been talking earlier. Now present was a hostile, snarling, bragging, cussing "person," interspersing his comments with four-letter words and claiming "credit" for having "done-in those broads" in Bellingham and in Los Angeles. Note that the Steve alter spontaneously emerged when the examiner focused attention on the headache and inner turmoil. Later Steve complained of the difficulty he had in "coming out."

Other signs of dissociation may be somatization reactions in various bodily systems, and true MPD cases frequently report hearing "voices in the head." These voices are usually different from psychotic auditory hallucinations, which are experienced as coming from outside the head (Bliss, Larson, &

Nakashima, 1983), and cannot generally be decreased or eliminated by medication.

Typically, MPD patients have had numerous previous diagnoses, such as sociopath, manic-depressive psychosis, schizophrenia, adjustment disorder, borderline personality, antisocial personality disorder, or some type of organic condition. They have often been hospitalized and have been evaluated at many clinics and by numerous practitioners, who disagreed with each other. This failure to diagnose correctly is especially marked when sufferers from dissociation arrive at the offices of psychologists or psychiatrists who do not believe in the reality of MPD (Koch, 1985). All this compounds the problems and distrust of the patient. He or she dissociated in the first place as a protection against abuse. Family and friends have not understood her, have often condemned her erratic behavior, and accused her of lying, even though she is being honest when she vehemently denies acts or words clearly heard by others. She commonly experiences this same disbelief in the examining room of the skeptical clinician, and interprets it as further abuse, but with the doctor now as the abuser. No wonder that the MPD therapist is confronted with a nonrevealing, suspicious, and hostile individual whose treatment will be time-consuming and exasperating.

MPD patients often report the unexplained loss or possession of objects, or the finding of notes which they had apparently written, but for which they have no memory. These notes may be in handwriting distinctly different from their own.

Sometimes depersonalization, the inability to experience their own self; derealization, wherein the external world does not seem to be real; trance-like sensations; or "out-of-body" feelings, that is, perceiving one's own body as external, "out there," will be revealed. Sooner or later the experiencing of much abuse as a child, physical, sexual or mental, will usually be reported.

Other indicators of possible MPD are sudden shifts in mood and voice and uneven achievement in school despite high intelligence (and MPD patients usually have high intelligence).

During switching from the host personality to an alter or between two alters there are often postural and gestural signs, such as eye rolling, shoulder twitching, head turning, changes in seating posture—and sometimes even petit mal seizures. The patient's manner is often inappropriately deferential, with an excessive need to please, suggestive of a child's attempt to placate a potentially abusing adult.

A number of objective tests have been devised, which can add to a diagnostician's armamentarium in delineating these cases. *The Dissociative Disorders Interview Schedule* or *DDIS* (Ross et al., 1989) is a structured interview designed to make differential diagnoses between MPD and a number of related conditions, such as borderline personality disorder, depression, and somatization, has been widely used.

Another significant test is the *Dissociative Experience Scale (DES)* by Bernstein and Putnam (1986). This is a brief self-report inventory of both normal and abnormal experiences designed to measure the extent of dissociative psychopathology. It has had a substantial number of studies investigating its validation, most of which have been very positive, and it is widely used as an initial screening test of potential dissociation (Anderson, 1992; Carlson & Putnam, 1993; Draijer & Boon, 1993; Ellason, Ross, Mayran, & Sainton, 1994; Ensink & van Otterloo, 1989; Frischholz et al., 1991, 1992; Ross, Norton, & Anderson, 1988.

Sanders (1986) has published the *Perceptual Alteration Scale*, constructed in conformity with Hilgard's (1986) description of dissociation. It consists of some 60 items that have been shown to distinguish between "normals," bulimics, and MPD.

A recent scale, which is getting widespread attention, is the *Structured Clinical Interview for DSM-IV Dissociative Disorders*. In its most recent form (Steinberg, 1994) it is called the *SCID-D*. This scale consists of some 258 items measuring the processes of amnesia, derealization, depersonalization, identity confusion, and identity alteration. These are related to the *DSM-IV* diagnoses of dissociative amnesia, dissociative fugue, dissociative identity disorder, depersonalization disorder, and dissociative disorder not otherwise specified. The usefulness of this scale lies in the greater specificity with which it evaluates individual aspects of dissociation and relates these to specific diagnoses (Steinberg, 1995). There are a number of studies to date testing its validity (Draijer & Boon, 1993; Frischholz et al., 1991, 1992; Hall & Steinberg, 1994). It promises to takes its place as a more detailed instrument to be used after screening by the DES.

Other tests which have shown promise are *The Phillips Dissociation Scale* or *PDS* (Phillips, D., 1994) and *The Child/Adolescent Dissociative Checklist, CADC* (Reagor, Kasten, & Morelli, 1992). Vanderlinden, Van Dyck, Vandereycken, and Vertommen (1991) have reported a large-scale evaluation of dissociation in the Netherlands using the *Dissociation Questionnaire (Dis-Q)*.

An accurate diagnosis of MPD is especially important in the arena of forensic practice (see Allison, 1980, 1982, 1984; Allison & Schwarz, 1980; Coons, 1991; French & Schechmeister, 1983; Lasky, 1982; Lewis & Bard, 1991; Ondrovik & Hamilton, 1990; Orne, 1984; Savitz, 1990; Watkins, J., 1984, to mention but a few of the reports on MPD and the law). Moreover, the diagnosis of dissociation will often be disbelieved by a skeptical judge and jury. Multiple personality flies in the face of common sense and of a basic assumption in jurisprudence, namely, that a "person" consists of one body, and one "mind," which is responsible for his or her behavior.

CHARACTERISTICS OF MPD ALTERS

Alters think, react, and behave in ways similar to what we see in covert ego states, which have been activated under hypnosis. However, they do so to a more extreme degree.

Since they are part-persons they exhibit a much more limited knowledge and perspective than a whole person. Their thinking is often child-like and concrete. Cognitive processes tend to be rigid and not easily changeable in the face of contrary logic. In this respect they are not only dissociated from the primary personality, but they are also often dissociated from intellectual processes, such as common sense.

The question may be asked, "When does the patient switch ego states?" The simplest answer is, "When it is convenient." Switching is a matter of energy transposition. One gets the impression that the situation is like an electrical switchboard, where the energy is diverted from one motor into another. But why? One may be talking to the primary or host personality when suddenly a new entity appears, different in manner and voice, and which may identify itself by a different name. For some reason, in our conversation with the original personality something was said that made it more convenient for the patient to switch. Perhaps we asked a question that the host personality could not or did not want to answer. It abdicated. Perhaps the energy available to the host personality at that time was depleted, and a stronger and more highly energized state was able to become overt and assume the executive position. Or perhaps the course of the discussion was such that the underlying alter was more highly motivated to emerge and communicate, more so than the host personality's ability to maintain the executive position. Therapists are often confronted with a switch to a different alter when the therapeutic communication is getting too "hot" or threatening to the patient, or to the alter that is currently present.

The influence of an underlying alter that seeks to emerge may be noted by a tendency or "pull," on the host personality. By concentrating on it, the "pull" is translated into activation of the alter responsible for it.

A patient with an underlying alter known as "Hideaway" was describing the behavior of the host personality when standing outside a tavern the evening before.

> Patient: She mentioned to me that she didn't want to go into the tavern, and yet she did. Something made her go.
> Therapist: Oh.
> P: Something was pulling her in. It wasn't me. I was telling her to stay out. She was going in anyway.
> T: Is there somebody else who could be doing the pulling?

P: Maybe Medusa's back again. [An early alter, which hadn't made an appearance for some time]

T: Have you seen anything of Medusa lately?

P: Marilyn [the primary personality] was mad at her husband today, but Medusa wasn't there.

T: Let's go back to the time where she is standing outside the tavern debating whether or not to go in or not. Can you go back to that time?

P: Yeah. Now something's been telling her to go in, and we're going to hear from that somebody–now.

[A new entity emerges] Ah, go on in. Be an optimist. Go on in.

T: Who are you?

P: Me? Why do you want to know my name?

T: Haven't you ever told me your name?

P: Uh-uh. Not going to.

T: Why not?

P: 'Cause I don't want to [resistance or fear].

T: Would I be surprised or hurt if you did?

P: You'd be a little bit surprised.

T: You told her to go in?

P: Hideaway can go to hell. I'm the one that told her to go in.

T: Well, where have you been all these weeks?

P: You just never called on me before.

T: Well–uh–are you Medusa?

P: Uh-uh. Medusa's not around. I've been around since the 18th of July [two months before].

T: What happened on the 18th of July?

P: Don't you know? Marilyn came back [to an unhappy marriage from visiting relatives].

T: And then you started in?

P: Uh-huh.

T: What makes you different from Marilyn?

P: I tell her to do things she doesn't particularly want to do, like going in taverns.

T: You didn't exist before July 18th?

P: Nope.

T: Why didn't you ever talk to me before?

P: I didn't feel like coming out until today.

T: How do you like being out?

P: It's fun. I'm glad you got me out of there 'cause I wanted to talk to you.

T: Let's get acquainted. I'm Dr. Watkins.

P: Oh, I'm Marge.

In this short excerpt we see the activation of a new alter when the therapist, noting a pull on Marilyn, asked for the source of that pull. Marge apparently was dissociated on July 18th when Marilyn returned home and had to cope with a hostile husband. Subsequent discussion with Marge showed her resentment at the husband and her strong determination to confront him—something Marilyn could not do. Marge was created to cope with a situation Marilyn could not handle. The reticence of Marge to identify herself is also quite obvious, demonstrating the resistance often encountered by a practitioner. It should be noted that although Marge emerged at this time, when the patient was hypnotized, she had been out previously and continued to become overt occasionally without hypnosis—in line with our criteria for a true multiple personality.

The greatest pain occurs when all components of a traumatic experience, perceptual, cognitive, affective, and behavioral, are present at the same time—a "complete" experience. Accordingly, the individual may employ dissociation as a protection by deleting only one or more of the above aspects. For example, an alter may have complete memory and knowledge of an early trauma, but it is disclosed with no emotion. In the complete sense it is not being re-experienced in the here and now. In psychoanalysis we call this *intellectual insight*. Too often therapy or analysis achieves intellectual insights but not those complete reorganizing experiences which result in a permanent loss of symptoms. In situations like this, emotional, experiential abreactions can be of great value (Comstock, 1986; Steele, 1989; Watkins, J., 1992b, chap. 4, 1995). The achieving of only intellectual insight gives rise to such jokes as, "After five years of analysis he still bangs his head on the floor, but now he knows why."

Frequently an alter may demonstrate great fear but be unable to remember or describe the original precipitating experience. The perceptual and cognitive aspects have been eliminated by dissociation. The therapist will strive to lift this dissociation and permit an integration in all spheres, recognizing that there will be resistance. The patient will experience much anxiety and pain, since it is precisely this "completeness of reexperiencing" that the dissociation was erected to prevent in the first place. The key to helping the individual surmount this point of resistance lies greatly in the close relationship the therapist should have established with the patient.

Even though achieving a complete experience, involving all perceptual, cognitive, and affective components, is usually a desirable goal when integrating a multiple personality, sometimes a limited therapy requires that we focus on one of these factors, the one in which the greatest conflict lies (Watkins & Watkins, 1993b).

Alters can be quite large with broad cognitive and behavioral potentials, almost complete persons, or they can be quite small with their experiential repertoire limited to a very specific situation. In such cases we may consider them as simply personality fragments, and not treat them as separate personalities. In treatment it may not be important to give them a great deal of attention at the expense of more significant ego states. As the entire individual becomes integrated these fragments tend to drop out or combine with larger entities.

Alters tend to be specialized in their function. Thus, one is the musician with the ability to play a Bach concerto while other alters are incapable of rendering "chopsticks." One alter may be the system's athlete, while still another is more of an artist. To outside observers the individual appears to be quite talented and to function at a high level in many activities. They do not realize that only a currently executive alter is functioning at the high level in that particular area. It is not uncommon that certain alters become jealous of the skill of another alter (or the attention it receives), and try to sabotage it, sometimes successfully.

Since alters think concretely, they frequently are not aware of the consequences of their behavior. One alter attempted to get the patient to drink poison, reasoning, "When she's gone, then I'll come out all the time and be in charge." When we recognize that alters are usually children whose reasoning has been frozen at the time they originated, their puzzling actions can be better understood. One may have much difficulty trying to reason with a four-year-old child. Clinicians often fail to realize this when confronted with an adult body. We have usually forgotten how we thought (concretely) when we were children.

Alters that originated in child abuse are typically guilt-ridden. Their reasoning is that they were abused because the patient was herself "bad," a point of view probably forced on the child by the abuser and accompanied by threats. In treatment, this layer of guilt needs to be dealt with, and it does not disappear through simple reassurance. Much reassurance over long periods of time by a trusted therapist may be required to make a dent in it. The therapist must realize that this need for a rigid, fixed belief, "I am bad and I am to blame for what happened when Daddy came to my room," is a kind of psychological glue that binds together the whole protective, dissociative structure. All the defenses of the patient may be mobilized to maintain it.

Dissociation is a fascinating phenomena that occurs much more widely than commonly thought. It can help children (and adults) cope with frightening situations, keep peace between contending ego states, and assist the self in surviving with more equanimity. It appears in out-of-body experiences, in dreams, and in countless ways in "normal" people. It is only in its severe manifestations, such as we see at the extreme end of the differentiation-dissociation continuum, that it becomes pathological. When very segregated ego states are created, behavior and perception is compartmentalized, and the price for temporary surcease from inner conflict and mental pain may be a severe mental illness, such as multiple personality disorder.

MPD alters interact with each other and with the total personality in ways which are both difficult and fascinating to trace. They often display interactions overtly that one sees in covert ego states, but only when they are activated by hypnosis.

The experienced and sensitive therapist can approach an MPD patient with much greater understanding if he or she is well-versed in the science of psychodynamics, a study of intrapersonal processes to which we next turn our attention.

5

UNCONSCIOUS PROCESSES AND PSYCHODYNAMIC UNDERSTANDING

Sixty-five years ago, in the heyday of Watsonian behaviorism, a "scientific" psychology seemed to be in close reach. It was all a matter of finding the appropriate stimulus to elicit the desired response. The professor teaching an introductory course in psychology would ask a student volunteer to sit on his desk. Then with a small mallet he would tap just below the kneecap of the subject, and presto, the leg kicked. Stimulus elicits response. He explained that this is the way behaviors worked, enlarging the point a bit to conclude that each behavior was caused by the appropriate "situation" (a term which included *all* the impacting stimuli).

This idea was very exciting to a young psychologist who wanted to know the technology for understanding and controlling people. Unfortunately, it didn't prove to be that simple. It seems that the stimulus has to go through some internal and not observable processes before emerging as behavior. One is reminded of an old song that was published with the picture of a tuba player on the cover. It went as follows: "You push the first valve down. The music goes round and around, and it comes out here"–pointing to the bell. Somewhere between the air on the mouthpiece and the sounds being emitted at the bell a lot of things were happening–processes working and changes occurring. Of course, if you knew what valves were being pushed down, you could accurately predict the sounds that would result.

Human beings seem to function similarly. You can stimulate them, but before the behavior occurs it is first modified by the "round and around," so that one cannot predict accurately what will emerge. And the in-between processes, including which valves are being pushed down (called "intervening variables"), often seem to be unobservable to either an outsider or the subject himself. They are "unconscious," a dirty word in behavioral science. How can you measure and understand phenomena when they are invisible? It remained to Freud and his followers to devise ways of getting at these intervening processes, so they might be managed. Thus began the discipline of *psychodynamics*, the study of the unconscious "round and around," (Watkins & Watkins, 1996b).

Psychoanalysis did develop procedures for accessing these processes, but they took such a long time. Hypnosis, although rejected by Freud, offered a more expeditious way of understanding the "round and around" and gave techniques toward modifying intervening variables, so as to help people become aware of their inner processes and learn to behave in more constructive ways. Accordingly, the treatment approach of *hypnoanalysis* arose from an integration of the concepts of psychoanalysis with the hypnotic modality.

Psychology implies "the study of the mind" in its original derivation. However, during the eighteenth and nineteenth centuries the physical sciences made such progress and achieved such prestige that psychologists wanted to redefine the area of their study.

Modern science produces its results by objective measurement of tangible elements, and its terms are transmittable (pounds, feet, meters, etc.) from one scientist to another. "Mind" is an intangible, and only indirectly through language can one person understand what is in the mind of another. Accordingly, psychologists, in their eagerness to be recognized as respectable scientists, began talking of their discipline as the study of "behavior," and classified it as a "behavioral" science.

Unfortunately, this perspective ruled out of consideration the vast amount of internal experiences that people have, and that are not always revealed through overt behavior. With less of a need to prove our scientific respectability, the following definition of psychology might be more appropriate: *Psychology is the study of behavior and experience in as scientific a manner as possible.*

Behavior and Experience

People manifest themselves in many ways, both directly and indirectly. We can see another person move in space (behavior), and we can indirectly infer what is going on within him or her by the person's speech. People have emotions (feelings), and sometimes through observation of their behavior we can deduce what they feel because of how we, ourselves, behave when experiencing the same feelings—hence after the fact.

Understandings and meanings are still less tangible and, hence, less subject to behavioral observation, yet they constitute much of the "content" of a person with which we must deal in psychotherapy. Behavior is greatly determined by our inner meanings and understandings, as well as our feelings, and therapy is tremendously restricted if we concern ourselves only with behavior.

Cognitive Behavior and Meanings

As psychologists increasingly realized that their discipline must study more than behavior, the region of intellectual or cognitive activity was added. Behavior therapists became cognitive-behavior, or simply cognitive therapists. Still, inadequate attention was given to the emotional and perceptual functions of humans, not to mention those that were below the surface of consciousness. Cognitive psychologists and therapists studied the responses of people through their conscious verbalizing, which could be overtly heard and objectively evaluated. However, it remained to Freud (1938) to open up the region of behaviors, perceptions, motivations, and emotions that occurred within individuals, that could not be directly observed by others, and by being "unconscious" were also not observable and reportable by the individuals themselves. That is the area we will be discussing in this chapter.

Interpretation

Almost all therapists interpret to their patients how they, the therapists, understand that person. Based on observation and theory they try to transmit to the patient a comprehension of that individual. However, so much of therapy today, even when supposedly based on psychodynamic understanding, is practiced by attempting to tell, suggest, or persuade the individual *consciously* of this understanding. The therapist may often be quite correct in the interpretation. However, if it is made only to the more external and conscious facade of the patient, the interpretation may not reach the deeper areas of meaning and feeling which influence much of experiential and behavioral change. The therapy goes on interminably, and constructive change in the patient, if it occurs at all, does so very slowly. The understanding is only intellectual; it does not achieve insight.

Insight

The achieving by a patient of a new self-understanding is called *insight*. Freud had reported that insight brought real and permanent therapeutic "cure." It came to be regarded as a cognitive understanding of previously unconscious memories and their meanings. If this is all the term means, then we agree with our behavioral colleagues (Franks, 1983) that this insight does not necessarily heal, and may not even be relevant to therapeutic progress. Insight, however, can be much more than awareness.

An insight that is only cognitive or intellectual is like an individual standing on a hill and viewing the perspective of his home town in the valley below. He sees the crooked streets, the neglected slums, the crime-laden areas, etc., and he understands the needs. But as long as he views this town from the hill only as an object out there, no change occurs. Through insight he knows that he is looking at himself, but it is like a picture of himself. It is an object, and not a real experience of "selfdom." He must descend into the town, *experience* it as a citizen, feel its pain, and become involved. The "self-town" must become subject, not remain merely as an object. Since it is "his town" he must *reexperience* it with his whole being, as he did "for real" originally as a child. To change something he must be "there," where it is. Insight must be much more than cognitive understanding. It must be a level of meaning that is experiential, affective, perceptual, motoric (as well as cognitive), involving every tissue of his or her make-up, physical and mental. It is a "gut" understanding as well as a cerebral one. Such *genuine* insight releases in the patient new reserves of vigor, because energy that had previously been employed in repression or dissociation is now made available for more effective living.

Patients who have achieved recent genuine insights often comment on how the trees are greener, the skies bluer, and how much stronger they feel in coping with their world. It is *this kind* of insight that heals and results from psychodynamic understanding. When defined in this way, insight is a very potent agent for therapeutic change.[1]

Examples of Psychodynamic Interactions

Careers often are chosen because of unconscious needs. For example, a long life of service in an occupation devoted to the care of others may sometimes stem from a deep underlying feeling of guilt, warranted or unwarranted.

A physician in hypnoanalysis discovered why he became a doctor. Once, at the age of 11, on returning home from school, his father scolded him for not washing the dishes. He retreated from the room, muttering under his breath, "Drop dead." Five minutes later the depressed father did exactly that by going to the basement and shooting himself in the head. Desperately the youth tried to staunch the blood, but was left crying by his dying father. He then worked very hard to enter and graduate from medical school, and devoted his life to saving others—who (unconsciously) represented his father. He had been relieving inner guilt in this way, since covertly he believed that his remark had caused the death of his father. His insight into this conflict during therapy enabled him to forgive himself, be relieved of a long-lasting, low-level depression, and enjoy life.

Children tend to think concretely and often have very sensitive psychodynamic understanding, a skill that is often lost when they become adults.

Reik (1957, p. 575) describes the following incident: A young man with his eight-year-old sister are observing a number of children playing games in a schoolyard. One of them, Elsie, who is obviously greatly admired by a boy named Lawrence, has been chosen by him to be the "umpire." Elsie is particularly severe on Lawrence, condemning him to be spanked by all the other children. Puzzled, the young man turns to his little sister, Daisy, and asks why Elsie is so mean to poor little Lawrence who was so nice to Elsie and admired her. Daisy replied, "She treats him awful. She likes him best of all the boys in town." How wise we are when we are children.

The study by therapists of psychodynamics is often a reacquiring of the more sensitive understandings out of which we grew in becoming adults. Psychodynamic understanding (concrete or unconscious thinking) is further discouraged in the graduate school training of psychologists. Objectivity and Aristotelian logic are emphasized so as to make good researchers, even though after graduation most psychologists enter clinical practice and publish little research. Medical practitioners and even some psychoanalysts suffer from this emphasis on scientific objectivity.

Sometimes slips of the tongue or changes in behavior, posture, and manner signal covert motivations. These are frequently recognized by others and are the sources of humor. A young man became aware of his underlying resentment at an older brother only when asked why he rubbed his neck every time the brother's name arose in therapy. He was greatly surprised to realize that his father's frequent expression to characterize a person the father disliked ("he's a pain in the neck") could be why his unconscious translated an apparently meaningless movement into a covert communication. The psychodynamically sophisticated therapist is aware of such possibilities and carefully observes "random" movements or changes in posture.

A defensive maneuver commonly practiced by people to deny or avoid responsibility for their aggressions against others is the displacing of energies from a piece of self and changing it into object. How often do newspapers report that the criminal in court showed "remorse" for his crime ("I am sorry that *it happened*"). This is done to elicit sympathy and perhaps a lighter sentence. The real meaning of the statement is, "I am sorry I got caught." If true remorse actually was involved, he would probably have said, "I am sorry that *I did it*."

Even as it is important to understand possible psychodynamic communications through sensitive listening and observing, the realistic therapist must avoid the other (all-too-often) tendency to engage in undisciplined speculation. The subtle cues one believes to have received may or may not be true, and analytic speculation based on theory should not be taken as validation of mere hypotheses, which must later be tested.

When interpretations are offered to the patient, one may find that they are initially accepted because they are true, or initially rejected because although true, they were not presented by the analyst with the proper timing and preparation. And sometimes, they are not true at all. The clinician should be willing to recant and not be defensive in order to maintain the trust of the patient. None of us are omniscient. Psychodynamic interpretations should be put forth initially in a tentative manner, not as a proven certainty. Falling back on a "doctor is right" attitude, when the later data does not support one, is a good way to lose one's patient.

Learning Psychodynamics

Psychoanalysts have been the therapists who have most studied and practiced psychodynamics in their treatment. Yet as one surveys the psychoanalytic literature over the years in the hope of acquiring analytic wisdom, one is struck by the paucity of published material in which a master clinician shares his clinical sensitivity in such a way that it can be read, learned, and practiced.

For example, in some psychoanalytic studies one is told by the writer, "At this point I interpreted the patient's negative transference." But we seldom discover just how the analyst knew that the patient had negative transference. Just why did the negative transference arise at this moment in the treatment? With exactly what words did the analyst make this interpretation? And what was the patient's immediate response? How did this interpretation affect the patient's behavior, feelings, experience, etc.? We are too often left with a thousand questions, since very few analysts record their sessions verbatim and then study in detail their own and their patient's responses.

Much attention is given to general concepts and philosophy. Thousands of pages in the psychoanalytic literature are spent arguing complex points of theory, such as, just what did Freud mean at this particular stage in his development?

Theoretical arguments range from the original Freud-Jung-Adler debates to the contributions of Rank (1950) and now to the more recent arguments between the classical "drive" theorists and the "relationists" within the object relation school of psychoanalysis (see Greenberg, 1991, Greenberg & Mitchell, 1983). These include the relative merits of differing theoretical contributors, such as Fairbairn (1952), Guntrip (1968), Hartmann (1939, 1964), Jacobson (1964), Kernberg (1976), Klein (1932), Kohut (1979), Kris (1979), Mahler (1975), and Winnicott (1958).

As "philosophies" regarding the psychological structure of humans, these contributions are valuable and interesting. Yet after all this discourse one is left asking, "Just how does a master psychoanalytic therapist produce results?

How does he or she think, and how can one acquire some of the same clinical wisdom?" There are a few of the old psychoanalytic masters who do share more intimately their thinking and psychodynamic understanding, the reading of which we found helpful in understanding our own patients, and whose contributions can be integrated into our more recent ego state conceptions.

Freud, himself, could write very lucidly, even though we read him through English translations of his original German. In volume III of his *Collected Papers* (Freud & Breuer, 1953) he presented five classical case examples: "Fragment of an Analysis of a Case of Hysteria," "Analysis of a Phobia in a Five-Year-Old Boy," "Notes upon a Case of Obsessional Neurosis," and "Psychoanalytic Notes upon an Auto-Biographical Account of a Case of Paranoia" (the Schreber case). These are all well worth reading for a therapist today.

Outside of psychoanalytic circles many present-day psychotherapists seldom read the original Freud. Yet these classic papers are good examples of Freud's psychodynamic thinking. One of the best and most enjoyable examples of Freud's analytic thought processes is "The Theme of the Three Caskets," *Collected Papers*, volume IV (1953). One can learn a great deal by studying these case examples critically.

In 1938 Freud described Theodore Reik as "one of the few masters of applied analysis." In *Listening with the Third Ear*, Reik (1948) shares intimately just how he does psychodynamic thinking, the specific associations that pass through his mind in analyzing an event. In *The Search Within: The Inner Experiences of a Psychoanalyst*, Reik (1956) supplies some of that which "is neglected in the study program of psychoanalysts." He compared this to "the musical term, ear training: the development of a higher sensitivity to musical phenomena of all kinds—for instance to minute distinctions in tones" (p. 393). And in *Of Love and Lust*, Reik (1957) describes with case examples his observations of the differences in behavior and thinking between men and women—observations that can be most helpful to the male psychotherapist who treats female patients, even though the traditional roles of women and men have changed. The reading of Reik's publications can be an interesting learning adventure for the practicing psychotherapist.

DREAM ANALYSIS

Other ways by which a therapist can develop an understanding of "round and around" processes are through the study of dreams. In fact, Freud once said, "The dream is the royal road to the unconscious."[2]

Dreams generally occur in light stages of sleep, when the vigilance of the ego is lowered (because it is less cathected), and repressed object material is better able to rise to the dreamer's consciousness.

According to Freud (1938) dreams represent fantasied wish fulfillments of unresolved strivings for pleasure. We are inclined to view them as the culmination in mental picture form of attempts at all kinds of problem solving. However, like other behaviors they do trace in disguised manner the "round and around" of psychodynamic interactions between original precipitating stimuli and their overt expression.

Freud noted four different intervening mechanisms: symbolic representation, displacement, condensation, and secondary elaboration. We might add to these all the other known defensive processes (such as reaction formation, denial, projection, rationalization) by which humans seek to avoid the mental pain of consciously and fully confronting their own unacceptable impulses. "Dream work," employing any of the defense mechanisms, translates original motivations into images that can be acceptably perceived—at least in a light sleep state. Through the tracing of this dream work process, we can understand better how these psychodynamic transactions serve to protect the individual from both inner and outer threats.

One can learn much about dream interpretation from studying the techniques of Wilhelm Stekel (1924, 1943, 1949). Although Stekel ultimately split from Freud, he was always recognized among psychoanalysts as outstanding in the field of dream interpretation. He developed and used his psychological intuition in analyzing dreams more than by the free association method employed by Freud.

In his many case examples, he followed a certain pattern: First, he gave the presenting problem and then a background of the case. Next he presented each dream with his (intuitive) interpretation of its meaning. Stekel believed that the initial dream usually portrayed the entire structure of the patient's neurosis, which would emerge during the coming analytic sessions. He reported a much shorter time for his analyses than did Freud and other colleagues.

The following is an example from the analysis of a physician patient I had several years ago. The final interpretation of the dream (verified by patient associations) illustrates the use of ego state theory in formulating its meaning.

The doctor, who enjoyed deer hunting, brought in the following dream: "I took my two young sons hunting. We drove the family camper. It was getting toward evening, and the fog was beginning to form. We were on a narrow forest road on the side of a mountain, straight up on one side and straight down on the other. I felt it was dangerous to continue on this course, so we pulled the camper to the side of the road, and I put blocks under the wheels so it couldn't go off the edge. Then we went to sleep. In the middle of the night I woke up (in the dream) to find that my littlest boy had gotten out of the car and was pulling away the blocks to the wheels. In great alarm I yelled, 'Look out, you damn fool! You'll get us all killed.' I then woke up to find myself (with great relief) safe in bed.

In a light hypnotic state the patient associated to many of the dream elements as follows: "The most noticeable aspect is my great fear. There was a real threat of destruction to me and my family. I always think of the camper as being 'the family' car." The patient previously had also used cars as dream symbols for women. There is, accordingly, some present threat to him, his wife, and his family. The threat is being activated by his "littlest boy," his most immature child state.

I asked whether there was any situation in his present life, perhaps in his practice, that might be a "danger" to him and his family. Sheepishly, he replied, "Well—I have a new patient, a very attractive young woman who has been acting seductively toward me. She really turns me on, and I have toyed with the idea of going to bed with her. Of course, that's pretty immature of me, because if it were known, I'd lose my reputation, my practice, and probably my wife and children. I've said to myself several times, 'Wake up, man! Get her out of your mind.'"

The dream appears to be a warning. He goes deer (dear?) hunting, but takes along his children (his child states, who are immature) to protect himself and his (family) camper he puts in "blocks" so that he will not "go over the edge" (falling for her and destroying his family). His littlest (most immature) state threatens to remove the blocks. He might "fall" (seduce her). The resulting fear overcomes the dream state. He "wakes up" in the dream, screams at his immature child state, and then really wakes up safely in bed.

In this dream, we see much interplay of psychodynamic processes between the underlying motivations—attraction for his patient and desire to maintain his reputation, career, and family. His conscious self had recognized the immaturity of his sexual desires here, and these have been repressed into a child state. This state now threatens to take over (become executive) and initiate "acting-out" of his impulses toward the woman. By awakening, first in the dream, and then in reality, he decathects the child state, and returns to his normal, realistic executive state, which will use common sense in the situation. The dream, when interpreted, gives him warning of the danger to himself and his family.

Hypnosis in the Study of Psychodynamic Processes

All of the techniques ordinarily used in dream interpretation[3] can be applied with the patient in a hypnotic condition. This often makes much easier the revelation of unconscious meaning. Hypnosis seems to be similar to light sleep in its lessening of censorship and uncovering of preconscious material.

It is like the relaxation on the psychoanalyst's couch, but with further extension into a deeper trance.

This same condition exists in hypnosis. The ego does not abdicate, as psychoanalysts have been taught, but it is less vigilant in its defensive stance, and unconscious material becomes more available to conscious awareness. This is the leverage which the hypnoanalyst can use in practicing a psychoanalytic therapy.

Psychodynamics in the Treating of Multiple Personality Disorder

Another learning exercise about psychodynamic processes occurs when an analyst or therapist first treats a case of multiple personality disorder (now called dissociative identity disorder). Experienced MPD therapists, after a period of getting acquainted with a patient, can often predict just which alters will emerge, when and why, because of their understanding of the particular psychodynamic patterns of alter-interaction within that patient. They also frequently know just which alter was responsible for some reported behavior or period of amnesia. Since the ego states (alters) can become overt through the inner motivational systems of the patient without having to be hypnotically activated, the therapist is offered much more direct insight into the internal "round and around" processes of the patient. As one alter abdicates and another appears, it becomes easier to fathom just what is going on and why that particular switch occurred. Ego state functioning becomes more understandable. In the MPD case we might not need to use hypnosis or classical psychoanalytic techniques, such as waiting for a transference toward the analyst to reach into unconscious processes, so as to understand and help our patient push "the right valves" down and move toward greater maturity.

Psychodynamic Interactions in Psychosis

Even as MPD alters overtly display psychodynamic interactions, psychotic patients often reveal their unconscious mentation in delusions, hallucinations, and psychotic verbalisms.

A paranoid schizophrenic patient once said to me (JGW), "We're trying to get a bill through Congress making General Marshall General of the Armies." It took some time listening to his symbolic equivalents before the meaning of this statement became clear. Congress, the nations's deliberative body, represented his own mind. General Marshall (the therapist), who defeated the Nazi evil (equated with his mental illness) brought peace to Europe through the Marshall plan of reconstruction (the therapy). Moreover, the first "General of the Armies" was George Washington, who was "the father" of our country. The patient was struggling to award to me a recognition of his willingness to accept me as a "father" for him, a new vote of confidence. I replied, "General Marshall is delighted to accept this honor." We have symbolically communicated to each other. I know that his "award" signifies a transference, which later may have to be resolved, but not until after his psychosis has subsided and he will be able to accept and integrate such an interpretation.[4] Of such is the nature of psychodynamic processes and their interpretation within an analytic psychotherapy.

It is time now to explore a severe case of dissociation to see how the different alters in a true multiple personality can interact psychodynamically with each other and with the primary personality.

6

PSYCHODYNAMIC MOVEMENTS IN MULTIPLE PERSONALITY ALTERS

Specialization of function through patterned segmentations, the dividing of a whole into parts, seems to develop for similar reasons in both individuals and groups. Initially, specialization is created for purposes of survival and adaptation by the organizing unit. If the part is successful in its protective mission, the whole develops more segments to meet other needs and problems. Policies that bring rewards and mitigate pain tend to be repeated.

Nations develop Departments of Defense to ensure their survival against external enemies. The severely abused child develops MPD alters to deal with the attacks of abusers. These are specialized segments originally established to cope with the problem of survival, and if the separating (splitting) procedure is reinforced, it will be repeated to meet less drastic needs, such as those of interest and pleasure. Ego states, both covert and overt (alters), proliferate and multiple personalities may come into being.

Within the normal and well-adjusted society institutions and agencies, states, counties, cities, and other governmental units cooperate and communicate first for survival and then for the enhancement of living. Optimally their activities are coordinated for the good of the entire nation, which efficiently meets both survival and other needs.

Within the normal and well-adjusted individual, ego states are differentiated for greater efficiency in living, but when confronted with extreme threat such as child abuse, they can develop overt alters with more impermeable boundaries, as in, for example, multiple personality disorder.

Unfortunately, when survival needs are predominant, the segments may cease to communicate or cooperate, and dissociation becomes the order of

65

the day. Struggle and competition develop. Factions within a nation compete for power. Nations war with one another. Corporations engage in economic battles. The "parts" erect separating "walls," and intra-unit communication ceases or is greatly restricted.

Within individuals a similar pattern can take place. Multiple alters, separated by amnesic boundaries, war with each other for the executive position within the entire personality. As in nations, control and territoriality are powerful motivations. The coping efficiency of the entire individual is seriously impaired.

Multiple Personality

A multiple personality is a system of equilibrium that strives desperately to cope with the many facets of a complex and brutal environment. It seeks first survival, then efficiency in living, achieves it to some degree, but so often fails. This striving is only a more extreme form of that in which the "normal" individual engages, who through differentiation (in a much milder degree of the separating process than dissociation) creates ego state parts designed to improve more efficient adaptation within a less severe social environment.

One of the most difficult tasks for the MPD therapist is the management of malevolent alters. When confronted with such entities the therapist may use one of many options. For example, he or she can try to *eliminate* the offending state, reduce its influence, and modify its goal to a more constructive one by *integrating* its efforts into the purpose of the whole, the entire personality. Sometimes this process means losing its unique identity in a *fusion* with the host personality or with other alters. Such fusion can occur spontaneously when the specific need or purpose of that state no longer exists. However, individual parts often strenuously resist being fused (Watkins, H., 1989).

This resistance within an individual is similar to an external conflict between individuals and groups or institutions. The army fights for its appropriations at the cost to other governmental departments even when a nation's need at the moment may be otherwise. The striving by parts may no longer be devoted primarily for the purpose for which they were created, the survival of the whole.

Parts may survive if they change and adapt to new conditions. Buggy-manufacturering companies survived when they began manufacturing automobiles. When polio was eliminated through the development of vaccines, did The March of Dimes go out of existence? No, it continued to employ its staff in the collection of charitable funds for the treatment of birth defects in children. Existence of an organized entity can be continued, even when the original mission for which it was created no longer exists, if that entity will change and adapt. In this manner the various alters in MPD and ego states in lesser disorders can escape extinction—a fact which can be used to reduce intrapsychic resistance and further therapeutic goals.

The therapist promotes this by expanding the thinking of MPD alters beyond their original rigid and concrete boundaries. And from the study of normal ego state problems under hypnosis we can learn much about tactics that are applicable with true multiple personalities. Let us consider some of the possibilities.

Elimination of Maladaptive, Malevolent, or Anachronistic States

The therapist, HHW (see Watkins, H., 1978), discovered a state in a non-multiple college student who came to treatment for obesity, which called itself The Young Minds. This entity (or group) reported, "We sit on the mind like ticks." They claimed to be "the fear parts" of the mind and reported they had been "born in the hospital" when the patient was very young. Helen asked, "Why were you born?"

"Because there was fear."

"Well, what is your purpose in being there like ticks on the mind?"

"We don't need a purpose; we only exist."

"Then you don't know what your function is."

"No."

Helen called for a case consultation with The Dark One, a previously malevolent ego state, whom she had befriended, and who now had been assisting as an internal auxiliary therapist.

"Hello, Dark One. You must have heard what the ticks said, those fear parts of the mind, as you heard them described. Uh, we need to do something about it. What do you think?"

She then asked if he could stop their activity, and he replied that he would be willing to try, indicating that, "it won't be easy." He then contracted to do the job in three days by "reducing their influence and cutting off their energy," but noted that during that time "she," the patient, would behave differently. "She may be cold, distant—other people will bother her."

He did complete his contract in three days, and the patient was much freer of internal fear. The decision to eliminate "the ticks" was based on the information that they were no longer functional. They simply existed as maladaptive behavior habits.

In another nonmultiple case, we (JGW and HHW) had been communicating with Toby, a child ego state in a student who had emerged at the time he was brutally beaten by a cruel mother. The patient's "Toby" was dissociated and repressed, taking all the spontaneity and vivacity of the four-year old down into an unconscious, covert ego state. Only a bleak, schizoid shell of a person, depressed and burdened with much destructive anger, was left behind. In this way the patient had "saved" the most creative and "alive" part of himself. This patient was not a multiple, but the psychodynamic maneuver of splitting and repressing a segment of self is one often performed by multiples.

It became apparent that the main patient needed the alive, creative, spontaneous parts of himself returned to him if he was to function as other than a drab, depressed, and angry person. The therapeutic strategy first involved the release, in several violent abreactions, of the fear and anger at the mother. Then, when the reason for the splitting and repression of the Toby state no longer existed in the here and now, we could eliminate that state and return its contents back to the primary personality.

The matter was discussed with Toby, who volunteered to relinquish his existence and "give back" these parts to the main personality. He said to us, "Because I love you I am willing to die for you." In the midst of an emotional good-bye session involving all three of us, little Toby was hypnotically put back into the main personality and ceased to exist.

The student regained his creative and spontaneous self. Later he went on to graduate training, received a medical degree, and became a fine doctor, characterized by spontaneity, vivacity, and the ability to give and receive love.

In the two cases above, the elimination of maladaptive or anachronistic ego states could be successfully accomplished because they no longer served any survival purpose to the individual, and the integration was done by the agreement of all parties concerned. However, there is usually much resistance. Most ego states or alters are not willing to take the "Sydney Carter" role and die for the welfare of the whole person, even though it would be "a far, far better thing" for them to do (Dickens, 1950).

Psychodynamics in a Complex Case of True Multiple Personality

Occasionally we have taken into therapy various research cases for which we have not charged a fee. These cases were carried for long periods of time, sometimes several years. Our purpose was to study intensively the functioning of ego states, both when covert and when overt—as in true multiple personalities.

This book is not primarily about the overt ego states (alters), those which are seen in cases of multiple personality disorder. As mentioned earlier, there are a number of excellent texts currently available on the pathology and treatment of MPD. However, one of the best ways to study a process (such as personality segmentation) is to observe it under its most extreme manifestations. Such personality segments can then be compared with those represented in the more covert states found common in normal and neurotic individuals—the intermediate range of the differentiation-dissociation continuum.

This chapter reports on such a case. However, it is not possible to present a complete rendition of the treatment: It was conducted over several years, often with two sessions or more per week. While all therapeutic goals were not achieved (she moved away), there was much progress, and the individual is now functioning in a relatively successful and integrated way with little dissociation.

Our aim here is to picture the kind of problems faced by a therapist in MPD cases, the many ways in which dissociation is employed as a defense, and the interpersonal relationships between the host personality, the alters, and the external world—their "round and around."

For the protection of the privacy of the patient and her family, all names and identifying circumstances have been changed, including the names of the alters. The salient features concerning her behavior, feelings, conflicts, relationships, and therapeutic interactions are retained. This brief exposition of a long and complicated case must of necessity be a presentation of crucial incidents in its development and treatment. The primary therapist was JGW, assisted at times by HHW. During one stage in the treatment several graduate students (whom we have occasionally brought in for training in research cases) assisted.[1]

THE CASE OF SUSAN

A 30-year old teacher, who was taking graduate courses, was referred to HHW for counseling. In her session with Helen it was revealed that she was a multiple personality and had severe problems that would require long and intensive treatment. Helen referred her then to JGW as a research case. Over the course of several years some 25 different alters appeared, some as continuous participants within her internal conflict, others very infrequently. The primary personalities were as follows:

Susan: The original and host personality. Housewife, mother, and teacher. Weak and frightened.

Marla: Does the homework for teacher. Strong, capable, friendly, and good-natured.

Serene: The teacher in the classroom. Somewhat more aggressive than Marla.

Marianne: 6-year-old child. Angry, hostile, and afraid.

Alan: Adolescent boy. Athlete and concert pianist. Only Alan could play the piano. If he abdicated, the piano playing regressed to "chopsticks."

Denny: Angry 11-year-old boy.

Elka: 12-year-old girl. Artistic minded. Decorates house.

Alena: Does housework. Good cook.

Roselle: Late adolescent. Flirtatious, promiscuous.

Lion-Mom: Possessive and protective mother of Susan's three real children, Hilda (age 12), Audrey (age 9), and Paul (age 5).

Chan: Young child (5 to 8 years old). Angry, behavior problems. Very concerned about issues of fairness. Hid under the bed (when out).

Christa: Twin of Chan. Timid, shy, depressed, and fearful.

Richard: Unknown "cellar dweller." Ruffian. Strong. Makes plans.

Marlene: Angry, impulsive, aggressive. Lives (psychologically) in "the cellar."

Muriel: A 13-year old trying to act like a protective mother.

The Other: Dark, sinister, silent, and threatening.

Other alters, which made infrequent appearances, included: Alessandra (delicate and sensitive), Moya, Little Girl in the Well (seen once), No Name or Melanie (enforces rules), Tara (keeper of the door), Millicent, Sonnie, Constance, Theda, and Johnnie.

After many sessions various alters revealed that Susan had been subjected to severe sexual and physical abuse by her father. Her mother was constantly "sick," passive, subservient to the father, and avoided seeing what was going on. Both parents came from respected professions.

The first few months of therapy were spent mapping the personality structure, the various alters, their purposes, attitudes, awareness of each other, and interactions with Susan. Particularly difficult were Marianne and Marlene, who when they emerged often tried to run out of the session, and even threatened the therapist. Sometimes the therapist stood in the door and faced down an angry alter, not permitting it to leave, and even physically restraining it if it attempted to strike the therapist.

In one particular session Marianne threw chairs at the therapist, called him vile names, screamed, and tried to run out of the room while the therapist barred the door. After a time, while being restrained, it abdicated and a more benevolent alter came out. At no time did the therapist strike back, but sometimes he held the patient's wrists to prevent injury to herself or to him.

At all times he expressed concern and caring, even for the violent, angry state. It was also important that the patient not leave the session with an angry alter in charge. At one time this was not prevented, and the alter tried to get Susan to wreck her car on the way home.

Twice Marianne threatened suicide or to go home and kill the children. Being much concerned, the therapist or one of his assistants drove immediately to the patient's home only to be confronted with a smiling Marla who had no recollection of the threats.

During this period a therapeutic dilemma presented itself. If the therapist thought the patient's children might be killed (or even abused) he was required by law to alert the authorities, in which case they might be taken away from the patient. However, it was quite obvious that if this happened the patient would commit suicide, and a family tragedy would still not be averted. Through arrangements with a local psychiatrist the patient could be hospitalized, but this usually resulted in a loss of trust and a setback for the therapy. So, generally, psychological methods of control were utilized, such as rapidly hypnotizing the patient, calling for a more constructive alter (or a group of alters) who would restrain the angry one, and who would agree to prevent suicidal or homicidal behavior. This maneuver was usually successful, but at times some of the alters would report the hiding of a knife or a gun—a situation which required remediation by the more constructive ones.

At one time the following "contract" was presented for signature:

> I will not take control of our body and then use it to attack the children, Susan's parents, Henry (Susan's husband), or anybody else or to do them harm. I have a right to be angry if I feel that way, but I will not threaten to kill or to injure any other person.
>
> If some other of our inside family takes control and attempts to harm somebody or threatens them I will use my energy and cooperate with all of the others of us to take control back and restore responsible behavior.
>
> In return, I expect to receive respect and consideration of my needs from Dr. Watkins and the others.

The contract was signed by Marlene, Lion-Mom, Alan, Denny, Samantha, Serene, Susan—and even Marianne. This did not include a number of the more angry alters. However, since it involved a pooling of the resources and strength of most of the major ones, the more malevolent states were kept in abeyance. They still were very angry, and there was the potential for violent behavior, but they were now more restrained, and there were fewer reports of the patient striking the children or threatening suicide. Sometimes it is necessary for a therapist to plan and accept temporary agreements and adjustments until inner fury in the more violent alters can be abreacted and released.

A therapeutic incident occurred during the second year that demonstrates some of the strange ways in which dissociation operates. It also illustrates how a therapist's best plans can go astray when dealing with a multiple. The patient had had several miscarriages. Alan told us that he had emerged during several of these pregnancies, and had "caused" the miscarriages because "men aren't supposed to have babies," and he was disgusted to find "himself" pregnant. He also reported much disgust whenever he emerged to find "himself" menstruating. For a period of time the patient had ceased to menstruate, and Alan claimed that he was the one preventing her. Later in the therapy, after Alan had received much recognition and acceptance of his masculinity, Susan resumed menstruation.

Lion-Mom had been present when Hilda was born, and accordingly Hilda was regarded by her as "her" child. However, nobody apparently was psychologically present when Audrey was born by Caesarian section, neither Susan nor any of the alters. The doctor had reported that there was no movement in Susan's body during the delivery, and neither Susan nor any of the alters admitted having experienced the birth. It was not surprising that Audrey did not experience birth-bonding to a mother. She was aloof, schizoid, and given to much internal fantasy. Could this relationship problem be mended or improved?

An opportunity came when Susan reported that she might have to have an hysterectomy. Marianne went into a panic and became very angry. She, Marianne, wanted a baby of her own, and now there might never be a chance. Our reasoning was that perhaps we could regress a hypnotized Susan to the moment of Audrey's birth, activate Marianne, and allow Marianne to experience the birth, thus giving her a baby and Audrey, a "mother."

Susan was hypnotized, regressed to just before the delivery, and Marianne was activated. Helen (HHW) was present with the therapist at this time and actively participated at inducing a reliving of the birth experience (see Watkins, H., 1986a, 1986b). The experience went well. Marianne felt the labor pains, experienced the Caesarian, and held "her" baby, Audrey. She was most happy, and we congratulated ourselves on a therapeutic coup. Marianne had "her baby," and Audrey would now have "a mother."

The next session, Marianne came storming in, screaming at us for having tricked her. She had gone home, and there was no baby there named Audrey. Instead there was a nine-year old girl, who wasn't at all the baby whose birth she had experienced. She was furious and "would never trust" us again. We had failed to recognize this contingency and let Marianne experience "her baby" as growing for nine years. The patient went through a period of destructive behaviors, and it took us many weeks before Marianne would once again trust us. This incident shows how easy it is for a therapist to fail to think concretely as does an ego state, especially a child one like Marianne. Manipulations of ego states can sometimes be helpful but require the utmost of care and consideration for all possible consequences, which in the case of multiples can be disastrous.

Multiples seem to have the ability to escape detection over many years, partly because others are skeptical (or shocked) at the emergence of alters, and partly because many clinicians do not understand multiplicity. Multiples learn to hide their dissociations to avoid censure and rejection and to respond in ways they think will be in line with the views of the doctor or other person with whom they are interacting.

Under regressed hypnosis Marla recalled the following incident:

> Funny, it feels right now as if I can't remember my own name. I remember the school principal standing over me, repeating over and over again "That is a lie. Your name is not Marla. Your name is Susan." So I learned to answer to a name that was not my own. I don't remember hating the name Susan. It was just that she was not me, and I was not her. I could not figure out why people could confuse us when the two of us were very different. I actually thought they were quite stupid. The change was so obvious. But it upset them all when I "lied" and "pretended" to be someone other than Susan, so I learned the rules of the game then.[2]

Several years before entering therapy Susan had been considered in her church as being possessed by Satan, and she was taken by well-meaning religious people to an exorcism. After several days of mutual praying and confrontation with "the demons," she appeared to feel better. She was then pronounced as "cured" and "saved." Within a few weeks her angry alters, who had merely been repressed, returned to make her life hell, which caused her to lose confidence in the church. Denny, Chan, and Richard were furious at the attempt to exorcise them. As a result, she had become much worse, and felt she could not trust anybody. A year and a half after this exorcism she described it in a letter to a friend as follows: "I am the woman who supposedly was 'delivered' of demonic influences. My life has been hell ever since that time. I cannot seem to sleep at nights. Nightmares, voices screaming—I would just as soon be dead than continue on this way." She then described in detail the many beatings and sexual abuse she had received from her father.

One should be very careful at attempting to eliminate any ego state, even a most malevolent and destructive one, since each came into being to "protect" an abused child, and has since constituted an essential element in the defense structure of an MPD's personality. We have made that mistake ourselves (Watkins & Johnson, 1982; Watkins & Watkins, 1988).

A better approach is to make friends with the angry alter, give it credit for having originally come to protect the patient, assume that underneath it still has that same motivation (which is now merely misdirected at threats that no longer exist), and teach it to continue its "protection" in more constructive ways. Misunderstood condemnations of alters as "demons" only make the patient worse.

It should be recognized that personality segmentation, even a severe one, as in true multiples, is not completely inefficient or maladaptive. Susan's alters each had a specific function, and during much of her life they effectively carried out their respective missions. Lion-Mom took care of her children. Marianne served as a reservoir for repressed rage. Alan played the piano beautifully and excelled in athletics. Muriel got her to school as a child and to the university as an adult. Roselle handled the sex, which a crude and uncaring husband forced upon her. Roselle originally enjoyed this function, and when she left there remained only a disgusting and painful memory to Susan, Marla, and most of the other alters.

Albeit with occasional breakdowns in adjustment, the "whole" person was able to cope with her world in a reasonably efficient manner. Of course, "border wars" often occurred. Angry little Denny would sometimes emerge when Marla was overly frustrated and beat up on Susan's children, of which Susan would not be aware when she later re-emerged. And sometimes when Susan was tired of a university class and "went to sleep," 13-year old Muriel would temporarily take over, trying desperately to take notes in the class from an instructor whose vocabulary was beyond her. Result: Susan might fail her next test, since she did not possess within "her" the course information needed.

Psychodynamic Displacements of Pain

A most interesting intrapsychic maneuver we have observed both with true multiples and with more normal ego state problems is how the subject deals with pain. The host personality or normally executive ego state will often displace a pain from itself to an underlying alter or covert ego state. The individual appears to have simply "turned off" the pain. However, we have found that another underlying state may have "received" the pain and will protest when activated. In one case the pain from a severe burn was displaced into a child state, who (unconsciously) screamed so loud that, to quiet it, an older adolescent state took the pain to itself—thus demonstrating the teenager's bravery. (We have discussed this further in another paper; see Watkins & Watkins, 1990b.)

There were times when a child state would become jealous of the attention Susan gave to one of her own children, even to the point of hitting the real child. Over the course of the therapy Susan learned that she had to love herself, her own child states, and at times hold and nurture them. As she did so, she became more affectionate to her own external children. This resulted in her son, who had become quite belligerent during his early grade school years, showing a marked change, moving from low grades to top of his class, and becoming successful in school sports.

This learning to love one's own self, and especially one's most unlovable and malevolent states, is a very important therapeutic aim. Often we try to find an alter that will take responsibility for, or take care of, one of the most hurt or lonely states. This *internal self-nurturing* is a technique very useful in all ego state therapy, but especially in multiple personalities, which usually have angry, abused, and fearful alters. How to implement this technique will be described in detail in later chapters.

Early in the therapy, Susan disclosed that many of the more angry "children" had been confined in "the basement." Later, when she felt stronger, a number of these alters rushed out of the basement into the first floor of her "house-self." This experience was very difficult, since it involved flooding herself with much of the repressed anger. The dissociative symptoms returned—sleeplessness, depression, and pain, plus anger at her own children (and sometimes hitting them). It is at times like these when the relationship between the MPD therapist and patient is most taxed—and is most vital. If the relationship is strong enough the ego strength of the therapist will be added to that of the patient and the pathological material will be handled, controlled, and integrated. If the relationship is not strong enough, the emergence of this material will have been premature. It will act as a new trauma, and the treatment will be set back. Much time must then be spent supporting the patient, while for the present that which she cannot handle is dissociated and re-repressed, awaiting the moment when the ego is strong enough to cope with it.

At times like these the therapist must cease probing, reduce stress on the patient, aid in the re-repressing, and work on strengthening the therapeutic relationship. Therapy becomes an alternation between lifting repressions, undissociating, and building the patient's ego, so that it can cope with and integrate new insights. Dealing with this necessary balance is the mark of the sensitive and skilled clinician. Estimating the ego strength of the patient and that of the combined patient-therapist interaction at each moment becomes crucial, especially in the treatment of multiples.

Therapists of patients with MPD must always take risks. No risk, no gain. But too much risk results in a therapeutic crisis, requiring disaster control before proceeding further. Treatment of multiples is not for the inexperienced, timid, or fearful therapist. The progress of MPD therapy is often marked by having it "explode" in one's face. When this is mishandled it can result in suicide, homicide, psychotic break, or violence to family members, not to mention civil suit for malpractice. As badly as they are needed, MPD therapists operate in a hazardous occupation. That is why an understanding of psychodynamics in general and of the pattern of psychodynamic interactions within one's patient is so important, even though never perfect.

Signs of Progress

Lest we focus only on the negative, there are many little signs of growth in our patients if we are alert to them. The dirty-faced, ragged little abused child alter may appear with face washed or a new dress. An adolescent alter may accept responsibility for helping a weaker one. Two alters, who are similar may decide to integrate into one. Nightmare dreams may be replaced with happier, constructive ones. Painful symptoms may subside. Greater success in work or school may be reported. The lessening or cessation of aggressive behavior against family members, and reports of increased abilities to give and receive affection may appear periodically in the course of therapy. The alert therapist reinforces positive behaviors and seeks to provide safety and understanding—rather than condemnation—when destructive behaviors occur.

Treating multiple personalities, even if only one, can be an entire graduate education in unconscious processes and psychopathology. But as one watches new growth in a pain-ridden, immature, destructive person and sees the unfolding of a happy, successful, competent individual, who can give and receive love, and who becomes a good citizen in society, the rewards to a therapist are great. As our dissociated patients become more real persons, so also do we, who share their therapeutic journey and participate in overcoming the problems, the hurdles, and the dangers.

7

EGO STATES IN THE
NORMAL INDIVIDUAL

Segmentation of the human personality can apparently occur at any point on the differentiation-dissociation continuum. At the extreme of the dissociation end, the compartmentalization becomes very obvious in the spontaneous, overt appearances of MPD alters. Less obvious are the separations that occur in the intermediate range. Their presence can be inferred by their influence on the primary individual, even as many unconscious motivations show themselves in transference and through other defense mechanisms (Watkins & Watkins, 1990a).

However, some form of hypnosis seems to be necessary if they are to be made overt and consciously observable. This suggestive focusing usually requires prior hypnotic induction into some degree of trance. Of course, good hypnotic subjects in psychotherapy usually require little formal induction. Simply an instruction to relax or "put yourself in a state of hypnosis" may be sufficient to bring about their activation.

The appearance may then be spontaneous (as in MPD patients who are not hypnotized) or it may require a suggestion such as the following: "Is there some part of Mary who knows what happened yesterday when she had the headache?" At this point a new ego state may speak forth.

The degree or depth of hypnosis required for activation depends on a number of factors, such as the trust and closeness of the relationship with the therapist, the length of time the therapy has been in progress, the mood of the moment, the severity of the problem that brought about the original creation of the ego state, and the hypnotizability of the patient.

Ego states, which are the product of segmentation when the original problem was severe and adaptation difficult, may require a lesser degree of hypnotic induction, even as true MPD cases may be said to be in a spontaneous hypnotic state when their alters emerge. In either case, hypnosis acts as a focusing agent and as a relaxation, which helps bypass[1] conscious defenses.

As segmentation approaches the normal differentiation end of the continuum, the pressure of these states to break through consciousness and become spontaneously overt is diminished. Accordingly, a greater degree or "depth" of hypnosis is usually necessary before they are made manifest. This, of course, lays the basis for criticisms we have received that ego states are simply artifacts created by the therapist through hypnotic suggestion. This criticism can be met by scrupulously avoiding the temptation to force a state to appear through excessive demands or seduction. The therapist or scientific experimenter wants to perceive what is there, not create an artifact.

The general principle is that these more normal ego states come about through adaptive segmentation by the personality in the solving of fairly normal problems of living, in contrast to the more severe, dissociative behavior manifested by the true MPD patient, who needed a drastic solution to a crisis, one often involving sheer survival. In the true MPD the excessive segmentation solves the immediate survival problem during abuse at the expense of suffering a severe psychopathology in later life.

Simple examples of normal ego states are demonstrated by the sports enthusiast who shouts, "Murder the bum!" at the ball game, while at home he is a withdrawn, taciturn person, noted for being unaggressive. All of us are usually in a different feeling state when working at an office than when at a party Saturday night. In fact, during the next week in the office we may not remember well what happened at the party. However, in line with experimental studies regarding mood retrieval of memories (Bower, 1981; Watkins, P. C., Mathews, Williamson, & Fuller, 1982), the memories of the happenings during the party may return at a time when the mood feelings of parties are again being experienced. From ego state theory we would say that the former ego state has been reinstated. This experience is in line with our studies of the "affect bridge" (Watkins, J., 1971), which will be demonstrated later in case examples.

The normal changing of ego states is also illustrated in bilingual people who have learned one language in childhood, but who now as adults reside in a different country and speak, often fluently, the new language of their present abode.

One of us (HHW) has had that experience. Born in Bavaria, Germany, she spoke no English before age 10 at which time (her father having died) she and her mother moved to the United States to live with an uncle and aunt in Pittsburgh.

The public school to which she was sent had no facilities for foreign-speaking students, and she was left to learn English on her own, as do small children first learning to speak. This did not involve the usual methods of a foreign language class, when a word in German is equated with the same word in English, for example, "baum" equals "tree." She simply created a new ego state, an English-language ego state, which learned the words as if for the first time, and she became quite fluent in English without a trace of accent.

When we traveled to Germany she spoke German to the store clerks, who took her for a native. However, this required a switch of ego states. When I (JGW) asked her to remember and tell me what month it was when she and her mother came over on the ship, she responded with "Juli" (pronounced "Yuli" in German). Her thinking had moved to a German-language ego state.

The same thing occurred at a dinner with some American friends in Germany. She was asked to translate the menu. With some hesitation she rendered the English equivalent of the items until reaching one which gave much difficulty. In a quandary she said, "I don't know what it is in English, but it is long, green, and you slice it." Her child ego state knew (covertly) the German word "gurke" but could not translate it (overtly) into the English "cucumber."

When asked during our workshop at a scientific convention in Konstanz, Germany, if she would present one of her lectures in German, she said simply, "I can't. All my scientific vocabulary and graduate training have been in English." Her German was spoken at the 10-year age level. This is a good example of normal ego state functioning, since she is not a multiple personality.

Sometimes people build a new ego state, and move permanently into that newer state which becomes the normal, executive personality, presumably repressing the original one.

A soldier in the American Army away from home noted that his wife seemed to be increasingly less interested in their relationship. At one time she wrote him stating she had decided to change her name from Louise to Jenny. During their next meeting it was Jenny who was present, and who seemed to have completely lost the previous love manifested by Louise. They were divorced, and she continued to lead the rest of her life as Jenny, even claiming a younger age. She, also, was not a multiple personality, but moved permanently from one normal ego state to another for some personal reason, and changed her life accordingly.

The Executive Ego State, Self-Concept, and Physical Appearance

When people look at one of us, they see "a person," an individual with certain physical characteristics, hair or hairdo, bearded or beardless, clothed in a certain way, etc. This is how our normal executive ego state appears to others overtly. They also see certain mannerisms of behavior, idiosyncrasies of speech, attitudes, and other personality characteristics that are generally stable and can be counted on to continue.

Accompanying these external attributes, which are visible to others, are internal feelings, beliefs, motivations, values, and other traits that together constitute who I think I am. This is my *self-concept*, and it also is relatively stable. It represents my feelings about my self.

When a different ego state receives the greater amount of cathexis and becomes executive, a new set of internal values may take place. I now define my self as different. Sometimes I feel like "a new person." At other times I may say, "I'm simply not myself today." Others may remark, "Henry acts like a new person. He is no longer depressed and withdrawn. Now he seems to be outgoing and sociable." This change may arise because a different ego states assumes the executive position.

During dissociation, an individual may have an "out-of-body" experience during which he perceives his body as external to the "self," behaving autonomously and not under self-control (as did General Schwarzkopf [p. 38]). In extreme dissociation, a true multiple personality may become manifested wherein one alter does not even know of the existence of a different one.

People whose executive ego state has changed may also alter their physical appearance as well as their attitudes, motivations, and values. Individuals generally maintain a certain constant external appearance, and that appearance often tells others much of who they are, whom they consider themselves to be. The businessman is seen wearing a suit. The cowboy sports blue jeans and wears his hat inside the house. Hippies, professors, the clergy often dress in ways similar to other people with whom they identify. This may apply to hair—its length, cut, etc. It may involve whether we wear a beard or a moustache, and whether the beard is neatly trimmed or permitted to grow without restraint.

When an individual dramatically changes this external appearance we suspect that something has also changed within. Perhaps a new ego state has taken over the executive position.

Many years ago, a depressed patient of mine (JGW), a middle-aged lady who always wore drab, dark-colored clothes, went through a significant experience in therapy. Her depression lifted, she proclaimed that she felt like "a new person," and she immediately bought a new set of bright-colored clothes. A different ego state had taken over.

When serving as a prison psychologist I (JGW) observed that many inmates dressed similarly. They wore their hair long, untrimmed, and sometimes braided down the back. They seemed to be making themselves look differently than "establishment" or law-abiding persons. By wearing their hair in this way they were demonstrating that they chose to identify with the other inmates, individuals who were, like themselves, in prison because of defiance of the law. Like the street gangs in Los Angeles who sport different colors, they were identifying themselves, their self-concepts, and their allegiances.

Often prisoners would appear before the parole board, avowing that they had learned their lessons, that they were changed men, that they should be let out of prison because now they wanted to be good, law-abiding citizens. Rarely did I observe one that cut his long hair, eliminated his braided tresses, shaved his beard, or in any way tried to look like the prison officers, who shined their shoes, cut their hair short, and trimmed their moustaches neatly. My thought then was, "This inmate hasn't really changed. He's lying about his 'new me.' He still identifies with his buddies, the other inmates." In fact, if he trimmed his hair, and no longer wore it like they did, they too would recognize the change and no longer identify with him or support or console him with "con" reassurance and bravado. If he had really changed, and no longer espoused their values, it makes sense that he would change his appearance accordingly.

I kept no records and have no validated data, but all too often those who remained unchanged externally remained unchanged internally. Their release to parole was only temporary. Soon they were caught in another crime and returned to prison. They had not really been rehabilitated.[2]

A prominent "Freeman"[3] in the West had become quite a national hero to the private militia, which are organized in many states to oppose the federal government. He had not made mortgage payments on his ranch, had refused for years to pay state income taxes, and would not get a driver's license or license his car. He had defied court orders and threatened law enforcement officers. Bearded, armed, and defiant, he challenged lawmen for months to come and get him if they dared, and when cornered fled to another state. During this time his ranch was foreclosed and sold at auction.

Personally well-liked in the community, he voluntarily returned months later and surrendered to law officials. He and his sons turned in their guns. Later, when he appeared in court, his beard had been shaved off, and he was wearing a conservative business suit. He was described in the newspaper as "far different in sounding and looking." Appearing before the same judge as previously, he agreed to all the conditions imposed, including the filing of income tax returns, and respectfully addressed the judge as "Sir."

He was charged with "criminal syndicalism" and "obstructing justice" and then released on $100,000 bail, put up by his parents. The judge, noting that he had agreed to be represented by an attorney, said that he and his family showed some "depth of sincerity on their part." When asked why he had surrendered he replied, "I intend to do what's right, because I do not intend to jeopardize the people who love me."

Many questions come to mind. Is this a real change of heart or is he only acting out instructions of his attorney in order to make a good appearance? Is this genuine rehabilitation? Has a new ego state become executive and taken over? If so, will it be permanent or will he revert to the violent Freeman behavior? What could have brought about such apparent change? Can love alter basic personality structure like this? In this case, only time will tell. But ego state theory does provide a rationale for such a transition.

Cases like these bring many questions to mind regarding the processes of change and rehabilitation in antisocial individuals. In prison populations I (JGW) saw many dissociated inmates in which whether a criminal behavior was carried out or not depended on which of several ego states was executive at a given time. There was often an alternation during which a criminal act was carried out by a hostile, malevolent, and angry ego state. Sometimes this state may have been replaced temporarily by a more benevolent one, one which could function quite well within the mores of society. Transformations like this may have resulted from a true MPD pathology (Watkins, J., 1984). However, in other individuals, angry, but more "normal" malevolent ego states temporarily assumed the executive position (Watkins & Watkins, 1988).

On the positive side, new ego states can be developed and incorporated that assume a more or less permanent executive role. This fact is obvious from many historical and literary examples. Saul of Tarsus changed and became the disciple Paul. Buddha, originally a playboy prince, changed executive states and founded a new, benevolent religion. And in the novel *Les Misérables* by Victor Hugo the galley convict, Jean Valjean, was rescued from becoming the "worst of men" and changed into becoming the "best" through the intervention of a kindly priest from whom he had stolen some candlesticks. The psychodynamics of this interaction are most eloquently described by Alexander and French (1946, pp. 68–70).

Similarly, the incorporation of a new and more constructive role model, such as provided by an interested policeman or athletic coach to a juvenile delinquent, has been well-known to change many lives. Perhaps it involves the introjection of a new, stable, executive ego state, whose content and role is more constructive. The potential contribution of ego state theory and therapy to such social problems has not as yet been explored.

Common Ego State Problems in Normal People

Covert ego states in normal people can sometimes cause transitory disturbances, such as anxiety attacks, psychosomatic pains, or interfere with behavior—such as with athletic performance. A former student of ours has been active in sports psychology, working with pitchers in a major baseball team. He has found that often when the pitcher is in a slump it is due to the interference of a covert state, which for some reason is trying to "punish" the individual. When the conflict was worked out in ego state therapy the athlete resumed his normal functioning. (Ritchi Morris, Ph.D., personal communication, 1985).

Ego State Resolution of a Normal Problem

Jill, a graduate student in psychology, was acting as an assistant in a class we taught on hypnotherapy. She was a good hypnotic subject and could demonstrate hypnotic phenomena; she was also a skilled hypnotherapist. During one demonstration she had emerged from trance, but was not completely alert and stated that she felt "spacey." Whereupon, Bert, a member of the class, said in a teasing way, "Well, Jill's always spacey." The class adjourned for the day. Later in the afternoon Jill called to report that she felt quite disturbed and was experiencing considerable anxiety. I (JGW) asked her to come to my office, and we resolved the problem with a therapy session. Jill felt that her experience would be valuable in training ego state therapists, so she came into the office the next day. The session was repeated and recorded as follows:

THERAPIST-PATIENT INTERACTION	THERAPIST COMMENTS
J: I noticed at the end of the demonstration I was feeling kind of dizzy, groggy, and I remarked that I felt kind of spacey. Then Bert, because we're friends and tease each other a lot, said that I was "always spacey."	(*Teasing is often common among graduate students.*)
W: It was kind of a facetious remark.	(*W trying to reduce impact of remark with reassurance.*)
J: That *was* a facetious remark. However, I found I felt rather angry at him. When I left the class I felt extremely agitated, very uncomfortable.	(*Accepted overtly but not inwardly.*)
W: You said it came about a half an hour later?	
J: I had a client scheduled, and I was so disturbed I had to cancel the session.	(*Inner disturbance quite severe.*)

W: All right, Jill, let's just do a hypnotic
   induction. [Jill raises her hand, is given
   induction suggestions, and soon relaxes
   into a fairly deep trance. After some
   deepening she is regressed back to the
   time just after her demonstration, when
   she was feeling upset.] You said you felt
   "spacey," and Bert made a facetious remark to you. After the class you felt in
   turmoil. Some part of you experienced
   that remark in a very disturbing way.   (*Regression to disturbing time.*)
   You're right back there. [Long pause]
   What is it, Jill?
J: I don't know you.   (*Surprising since J has been an*
W: You don't know me? Have you ever   *assistant in W's class.*)
   talked to me before?
J: I know Helen, but I don't know you.   (*J had been Helen's client.*)
   I'm not afraid of you, but I wanted to
   talk to Helen.
W: Well, you can talk to Helen later, but   (*W attempts to get J's trust.*)
   I'm Helen's husband, and she knows
   I'm talking to you.
J: That man. That man.   (*Bert not "a friend" or even*
W: What man?   *known by child ego state, which*
J: That man. He said a mean thing. He   *refers to him as "that man."*)
   said I was spacey or something, and I
   was trying to be a good girl.
W: That wasn't fair for him to say that.
J: No! Why did he say that?
W: Did you feel a little vulnerable when
   he said that?
J: I don't know what that means.   (*"Vulnerable" is a big word for*
W: That means you don't have any pro-   *child ego state.*)
   tection, like when somebody hits you
   and you don't have your hands up to
   protect yourself.
J: It felt like he hit me, and it hurt.   (*Child state had strong reaction to*
W: Was it a bad thing to say?   *Bert's remark, but wants to*
J: Yes. He was mean and dumb, and I   *please Helen.*)
   was just trying to be a good girl 'cause I
   knew Helen would like that.

W: How old are you?

J: I don't know.

W: What would you like to say to that man?

(W encourages a symbolic confrontation with "that man" to help J get a feeling of strength.)

J: I'd tell him he shouldn't do that. It was dumb to say that.

W: Let's pretend he's right over at that side of the room there. Look over there and tell him what you think of him.

J: Don't do that! It's not nice. I don't like you. Leave me alone.

W: You were trying to be a good girl, and the people liked you. Can I call you Jill? Is that your name?

(Reassurance to J following confrontation.)

J: No that's *her* name.

W: Whose name do you mean?

J: Her.

("Her," not "me.")

W: You mean the big one? Do you have a name?

(The big Jill.)

J: I'm the little one.

(Identifies self.)

W: Can I call you "Little One" then?

J: Okay.

W: I'd like to be your friend.

(Seeking to improve trust.)

J: You don't think I'm dumb?

W: Not at all. I think you were a very good girl, a bright girl, and everybody there liked you. Will you open your eyes and look at me?

J: No. 'Cause if I do that then she comes back, and I go away.

(Little One is a covert state. She is "out" only when under hypnosis.)

W: You don't have to look at me. Tell me about yourself.

J: Well, I like toys, and I like colors.

W: What's your best color?

(W trying to resonate more to child state.)

J: I like red. She likes bright things. She has something you hold up to the light and turn it around, and it makes colors. Do you have toys?

(Kaleidoscope.)

W: I used to have a little toy train that went round and round. Do you have a doll?

J: I have a teddy bear. His name's Teddy.

W: That man. Shall we tell him not to say   (*Bringing her to the problem.*)
anything like that anymore?

J: Yes. It's not right.

W: She's friends with him. We don't
want to get her into any trouble, do we?
She said she got upset after the hypnosis. Was that you?

J: I don't come out. I'm the one who
goes into hypnosis. She doesn't know
how.   (*Interesting.*)

W: I see. She's the one that can hypnotize other people, but she can't go into
hypnosis herself. Is that right?

J: I guess so. I'm not around when she   (*Clarification.*)
hypnotizes other people.

W: Do you give her a headache?   (*Little One now reports the pres-
J: Sometimes when she's boring. She's got   ence of headaches in J.*)
this thing with keys I don't know what   (*Computer. J is writing a disserta-
you call it. Sometimes when she does   tion.*)
that I give her a headache.

W: Does she know why she's got the   (*Headache occurs when Little One
headache? Does she know that you give   is bored. J is not conscious of this.*)
it to her?

J: I don't know.

W: Well, Little One, you can go wher-   (*How to dismiss an ego state.*)
ever you need to go, and I want the big
Jill to come back.

J: Good-bye [In a weak voice. Long
pause. Jill gradually stirs and opens her
eyes].

W: Hi.

J: Hi.   (*J no longer in hypnosis.*)

W: Well, what happened?

J: I feel better. I guess the regression   (*Disturbance reduced. Session was
made me better.   therapeutic.*)

W: I did talk to the Little One. You
know about her?

J: Yes.

W: She also said she would want to talk
to Helen. She knows Helen better

than me. We're going to let her talk
with Helen now. [Session termi-
nated.]

Jill is aware of Little One. She is apparently not aware of the source of her headaches when Little One gives them to her. Jill can hypnotize and do hypnotherapy. Only Little One, but not Jill, can go into hypnosis. Jill is a perfectly normal person, currently a college professor, and functioning at a high professional level. She is not a multiple personality.

The Hidden Observer

Hilgard hypnotized a demonstration subject in a class at Stanford University and suggested deafness. A student suggested that the individual might be hearing at some level, whereupon Hilgard told the subject that, even though he was hypnotically deaf, he might be hearing at some level, and if this was the case to signal by lifting the index finger. The finger rose.

Hilgard then repeated the experiment using anesthetic suggestions to cold-pressor pain instead of hypnotically suggested deafness. This involved hypnotically anesthetizing a hand and then placing it in circulating ice water. He found that often, even though the subject consciously reported no pain, a finger signal indicated that the pain was being experienced somewhere by some part of the subject. He held that this something was an underlying "cognitive structural system." He termed it "the hidden observer" (Hilgard, 1977, 1986). The experiments were repeated using ischemic pain, in which a tourniquet is applied to reduce blood circulation in the upper arm.

Hilgard regarded the hidden observer as "merely a metaphor or convenient label for the information source tapped" and not a "secondary personality with a life of its own." It occurred to us that perhaps his hidden observers were the same phenomena as the ego states with which we had been working. Accordingly, we replicated parts of his study for hypnotically induced deafness and hypnotically induced anesthesia to cold-pressor pain, using his verbalizations for making the suggestions. As subjects we used patients who had once been in ego state therapy with Helen, and whose major ego states were known to us.

When we activated hidden observers using Hilgard's verbalization, and then inquired about them further, we found different ego states, many of whom we had observed in therapy. Perhaps this can be best illustrated by reproducing here some verbatim excerpts of one such case (Watkins & Watkins, 1980).

AN EGO STATE THERAPY CASE AND ITS HIDDEN OBSERVERS

Ed was in therapy for a number of psychosomatic complaints. He could also apparently dissociate, since his wife reported that when he was absorbed in study, not only did he not hear her, but he also did not feel pain when she stuck him with a pin. In therapy he was found to possess a number of ego states, especially a "super-ego" entity, called Old One. Old One demanded that he constantly study and do everything "rational"—no foolishness. Ed was not a multiple personality, since none of his ego states emerged spontaneously. They could be contacted only under hypnosis. This session starts with Ed in hypnosis and Helen asking for the Old One.

THERAPIST-PATIENT INTERACTION

THERAPIST COMMENTS

H: And now I'd like to talk to the Old One. What's been going on?

E: It was a bad thing. It was trying to make me be bad.

("It" means object, a non-self force not under control of Ed or Old One.)

H: What was trying to make you bad?

E: Be irrational.

H: What does that mean?

E: Act irrationally. Screaming and hollering and jumping up and down.

(To Old One anything irrational is bad. He considers childish expressions of feeling irrational.)

H: He doesn't have to yell and scream, but he has to do something with those feelings. He needs to deal with them, and you and I made an agreement, if you remember.

E: You made an agreement with Old One. You didn't make an agreement with me.

(Uh-oh. A new one is executive, and Old One has abdicated.)

H: Oh, I thought I was talking to the Old One. Who am I talking to. Ed?

E: No.

H: Is it Omega?

E: No.

(H names a number of ego states she has contacted before in Ed.)

H: Is it Freak?

E: No.

H: Who is it?

E: I'm not going to tell you [voice of a little boy].

H: I'm not going to hurt you. What name would like me to call you? (*H reassures.*)

E: I don't really have a name. (*We don't give names.*)

H: How old do you feel?

E: I'm not very old. I'm older than you. Let me think now. I'm three. (*Not to be put down. Wants to appear big.*)

H: Oh, I like three-year-old boys. You must be lots of fun. You just want to be heard, don't you? (*H resonates.*)

E: Yeah, you talk to everybody else, but you never talk to me.

H: I just didn't know you were there. But now I know you're there I'm going to talk to you more often. (*Begins to secure his trust.*)

E: Oh, good. I don't have much fun.

H: What would you like to call me? Do you want to call me Aunt Helen? (*Good try, but a mistake.*)

E: No. Aunts are no good. All they do is knit and stuff.

H: You can just call me Helen, okay? You and I will play together.

E: [Wistfully] Will you be my friend?

H: I'll be your friend. You have a name for me; what shall I call you?

E: You can call me Sandy. (*He now trusts her with his name.*)

H: Okay, Sandy. I'll talk to you again. Will you step aside? I want to talk– (*Sandy protests at being left so soon.*)

E: I don't want to.

H: I'll talk to you later. Now I want to talk to the Old One again. I see a little three-year-old. Did you see him? (*Old One returns.*) (*Old One not aware of Sandy.*)

E: No.

H: We had a kind of agreement that I would teach him how to handle his angers in a constructive way. Okay?

E: In a constructive, *rational* way. (*Old One's rigidity.*)

H: You can't punish him with illness. Give him a little out. Now I'm going to count up to five. Coming up at the count of five: 1, 2, 3, 4, 5. (*He suppresses play needs of Sandy, and Ed gets "sick."*)

Ed emerges from hypnosis feeling relaxed. Many surprising interactions occurred between Ed's various ego states, one most noticeably. Ed had reported unable to concentrate on his studies in a foreign language course and was failing in it. Old One was very upset. Sandy emerged and said he was the one who had been disturbing Ed's study habits. If he, Sandy, was not permitted to play he would not allow Ed to concentrate. I (HHW) asked Sandy not to bother Ed during the day, but instead to play in his dreams at night, and Sandy agreed. In the next session Ed reported he had studied well, and in fact had gotten an A on his final exam. However, he was wondering why he had such vivid dreams every night, and in "technicolor." When Sandy was activated he said he had left Ed alone in the daytime but, "I've been playing at night instead."

HIDDEN OBSERVERS: PAIN AND DEAFNESS

In a previous study (Watkins & Watkins, 1979–80), hidden observers activated in ten student volunteers using Hilgard's verbalizations behaved like the ego states with whom we had been working in therapy. In the following study we activated hidden observers posthypnotically in a similar manner with five former ego state therapy patients, first with hypnotic anesthesia for cold pressor pain, and second with suggested hypnotic deafness. The following is a verbatim excerpt from the reactions of one of these, Ed (the previously described ego state case), in an experimental follow-up a year later. The experimenter is JGW.[4]

THERAPIST-PATIENT INTERACTION

J: Take your left hand and put it in the ice water. Hold it until it hurts too much. Then take it out. . . . Now I want to hypnotize you.

    [Ed is now hypnotized, reaching a deep state in some two minutes.] Listen carefully. I will take your right arm and hold it here, and it is going to become anesthetized. It will feel just like a block of wood. No feeling. No sensation whatsoever. You can't feel heat, you can't feel pain, and it will feel that way, as if *it wasn't there*, until I touch you on the shoulder. Coming up now at the count of five: 1, 2, 3, 4, 5. Now I want

THERAPIST COMMENTS

(*Ed holds hand in ice water for 15 seconds.*)

(*During this time Ed is holding his right hand in the ice water.*)

(*Note the words, "it wasn't there."*)

(*Ed is asked to pay attention to*

you to look at that picture there and describe it.

the picture to distract him from watching his hand.)

E: Sure. There's a couple of people on a sidewalk. There's an old lady with a cane and a girl with something. And there's a car with a guy driving it.

J: Look just at the little things and describe them.

E: I'm getting very dizzy, very sick. [At this point, I remove Ed's hand from the ice water. Ed has kept his anesthetized right hand in the ice water for 65 seconds as compared to only 15 seconds for left hand, prior to hypnoanesthesia.]

(Ed emerges from hypnosis.)

J: Okay. You're all right.

E: Oh, my stomach.

(Pain displaced to stomach.)

J: Your stomach is okay. I'm going to take the pain out of it. All the pain's gone now.

(Simple hypnotic suggestion to remove pain.)

E: That was really strange.

J: Do you have feeling in your hand or arm?

E: No.

(Posthypnotic anesthesia.)

    [Ed is now rehypnotized and asked the following questions.]

J: A few minutes ago Ed did not feel pain in his right hand. Is there a part that did feel the pain? If so, lift the finger of your right hand. I want to talk to you. Please come out, and when you're ready say, "I'm here."

(Hidden observer activated. Is it an ego state, perhaps one we already know?)

E: I'm here.

J: Who are you?

E: I'm the Old One.

(It is an ego state, Old One.)

J: What did you feel about the hand?

E: *It wasn't there.*

(Repeats previous words of J's suggestion.)

J: What do you mean, "It wasn't there?" But you said you felt the pain.

E: In my stomach.

J: How did it come that the pain was not in the hand, but you felt it in your stomach?

E: I was afraid.

J: Ed didn't seem to feel any pain in his hand. When I said, "Is there some part that felt the pain," you came out. Is that correct? *(Old One felt the pain, but displaced it from Ed's hand to his stomach.)*

E: Yes.

J: Thank you very much, Old One. Is there any other part of Ed that felt the pain in that hand when it was in the ice water? If there is, lift the finger of the left hand. [The finger lifts.] Okay, Part, would you come out and say hello? *(What about Sandy? Did he also feel the pain?)*

E: Hello.

J: Hello. Who are you?

E: [Mumbling] I'm Sandy.

J: Sandy, did you feel the pain in Ed's hand?

E: It hurt! What do you expect? Jeeze. *(He did feel the pain like a three-year-old.)*

J: Ed didn't seem to feel the pain.

E: Well, I did, and I didn't like it at all. Where's Helen?

J: Helen can't come right now.
  [Ed is now brought out of hypnosis, and his alertness tested. Then he is re-hypnotized.]

J: Listen carefully. When I count to three you will become stone deaf until I touch you on the shoulder. Coming up at the count of 3: 1, 2, 3. [The experimenter shouts "Ed" into Ed's ears and then claps two boards behind his ears. Ed shows no sign of response.]

E: I'm still not alert.

J: Hello, Hello.

E: I can't hear you.

J: You watching me talk to you? Hello? [Ed looks very puzzled. He reaches over and strikes the chair twice to see if he can hear in spite of his apparent deaf- *(Self-testing of deafness.)*

ness. When asked to lift a finger if a part
of him can hear, the finger rises.]

(*A hidden observer is activated.*)

J: Part, you signaled that you could hear
me. Are you a part that can hear?

E: [Faintly] I can hear you.

J: Yes, who are you?

(*We expect the Old One.*)

E: The Old One.

J: You're the Old One. Ed didn't seem to
hear anything, but you heard me. Is
that correct?

E: That's correct.

(*Old One confirms.*)

J: If there is any other part that heard me,
would you lift a finger? [The finger lifts.]
Would you please come out, and and
when here say, "I'm here."

(*We expect Sandy.*)

E: Okay.

J: Who are you?

E: I don't know.

J: Have I ever talked to you before?

E: No.

(*To our surprise, it's not Sandy.*)

J: Do you have a name?

E: No.

J: Could you hear me though?

E: I can hear you.

(*Another hidden observer ego
state. This was unexpected.*)

J: What's your name?

E: I don't have a name.

J: Where did you come from? Tell me
about yourself.

E: I've never been surfaced.

(*We have never used the word
"surfaced."*)

J: You've never been surfaced before. Did
you ever talk to Helen?

E: No.

J: Have you been able to hear what Ed
says and does all the time?

E: Yes.

(*Inner audition.*)

J: Do you play any part in his feelings or
behavior?

E: I hide things.

(*Unexpected.*)

J: You hide things. Does he know about
you?

E: No.   (*Covert behavior* [*unconscious*].)
J: Did you ever come out?
E: No.
J: Never before?   (*First time "surfaced," i.e.,*
E: No.   *executive.*)
J: Who do you hide things from?
E: Ed.
J: What kind of things have you hidden?
E: Things he doesn't want to hear. Who   (*An unconscious defense of Ed.*
    are you?   *Surprising, spontaneous reaction.*)
J: I'm Dr. Watkins. Do you know me?
E: No.
J: Did you hear me talking to you when
    Ed was deaf?
E: Yeah.   (*Confirms hidden observer*
J: Does it seem strange talking to me?   *reaction.*)
E: I've never talked before.   (*Interesting, but of course.*)
J: You've never talked before. You can go
    back down. Way down. Now, I'd like
    to talk a moment to Sandy. Sandy, can
    you come out?
E: Sure.
J: Sandy, a little while ago Ed was deaf. I
    shouted his name and clapped, and he
    didn't seem to hear it at all. Did you
    hear it?
E: No. Did I hear it? Was I supposed to? (*Sandy did not hear.*)
    Was it a joke, and I didn't get it?
J: Alright. Sandy you don't have to.
    You're a pretty nice boy. I like you.
E: Thanks, I like you. You're neat.   (*Spontaneous child reaction.*)
J: In a moment I want Ed to come back,
    and when he does, he'll feel good all
    over.
    [Ed is brought out of hypnosis.]
E: I'm really curious. Just for my own   (*Ed unconscious or amnesic to deaf*
    benefit, what exactly happened? Nor-   *experiment.*)
    mally I can remember everything.[5]

It appears that Hilgard's hidden observers represent the same class of phenomena as the ego states with which we have been working in therapy. Under

hypnosis they seem to be like covert multiple personalities, part-persons, each one with specific functions and limited behavior repertoire. They represent themselves as subject, hence, with individual identities, "I" or "me," and they perceive each other and the entire person as objects, "she," "he," or "it." Their spontaneity and unpredictability appear to make them more than behaviors elicited through demand characteristics, since they so often manifest reactions quite different from therapist expectations or requests. The recognition of the existence of such entities in normal individuals has significant implications for human personality theory and therapy.

8

PRINCIPLES OF EGO STATE THERAPY

Ego State Therapy has been receiving increasing attention recently, and a number of contributors have published papers on this approach (Edelstien, 1982; Frederick, 1993, 1994; Frederick & Kim, 1993; Frederick & McNeal, 1993; Frederick & Phillips, 1995; Gainer & Torem, 1993; Klemperer, 1968; Malcolm, 1996; Malmo, 1991; McNeal & Frederick, 1993; Phillips, 1993, 1994; Torem, 1987, 1993).

Ego state therapy is the use of individual, group, and family therapy techniques for the resolution of conflicts between the various ego states that constitute a family of self. The ideal internal status quo is that of cooperating units of personality. Even though there may be differing attitudes or needs expressed by these units, a democratic relationship between parts creates the least stress to the total personality. The treatment goals of ego state therapy are similar to those used by clinicians in dealing with true multiple personalities (Kluft, 1994). However, when dealing with covert ego states hypnosis is generally required to access them, which is not always necessary when treating overt MPD alters.

Human beings normally have mixed emotions, contrary needs, and are subject to the pull of outside forces. Such is the process of living. However, when internal states are sufficiently formed so that they have an identity of their own, as well as an identity with the whole individual, and in addition are rooted in the thinking of childhood, then conflicts are not so easily resolved. The degree to which an ego state will maintain its own identification will depend on the rigidity of the boundary that separates it from other such states or from the entire personality. In multiple personality disorder the boundaries separating the various alters are very rigid and impermeable; therefore, the resistance to change and the struggle to maintain its own individual identity by each ego state (alter) will be greater.

96

Childhood thinking is concrete thinking. It is literal and it springs from limited life experience. Furthermore, if an ego state arises through trauma, then the rigidity of thinking becomes even more manifest and thus harder to change by simple suggestion.

Conflict resolution may be the ultimate goal, but the route to achieving that goal can be more complex than suggested by this definition. Ego states have much at stake not to change their attitudes or behavior. Sometimes that stake, in the opinion of the ego state, has the magnitude of life or death, even though the executive state and the therapist may view the attitude as totally invalid in terms of the reality of the here and now. Changing such attitudes and behaviors, for the good of the total personality living in the present, requires both skill and art.

Most psychological theories seem to agree that human beings have a tendency to replicate the past, whether that past was happy or miserable. Whatever happened in childhood, we anticipate the same to happen in the present, even if we are not consciously aware of that expectation. Perhaps we want to change in the present whatever was not changeable in the past. But of course, such an anachronism cannot be accomplished. The timing is all wrong. But we try to do it nonetheless. Attitudes and feelings can change about past events but not the event itself. Therefore it is useful for the therapist to look for such misplaced patterns.

The woman who marries one alcoholic after another is very likely to have had a father who was an alcoholic. She tries to change each one without success, so that she can redo that painful past and have the father she always wanted. (One patient of ours was married to her eighth alcoholic!) No person would do such a behavior consciously, because it seems so foolish. To make sense, it has to be an unconscious process.

Further confusion and irony may occur if the wife is able to persuade her husband to stop drinking. She may be satisfied at first, but eventually the unconscious process of "getting him (father in transference) to stop drinking" takes over and she behaves in ways that promotes the husband's drinking. Unless the ego state contained in the trauma is healed, this circular syndrome may continue ad infinitum.

If the patient is transferring the past into the present, then he or she is likely to make that transfer into the therapy hour as well, which is a way of maneuvering the therapist to act in ways that were familiar from the patient's past.

Transference

The phenomena of transference has been well studied, and is the most powerful psychoanalytic technique (Freud, 1938). It is a simple but basic process.

Humans tend to perceive present figures in their life and to react to them as if they were former significant individuals in their lives, such as father, mother, sibling, teacher, etc.

The current individual is endowed unrealistically with characteristics of the earlier person. Thus, the patient may begin to feel that the analyst is uncaring and manipulative of him, even though the treating one has only been sitting and listening passively to the patient's memories. The analyst is eagerly watching for such a reaction, and at the appropriate time makes a "transference interpretation." He or she demonstrates to the patient that the analyst has not been manipulative, and that therefore the patient's feeling about this must have come from some other source. The analyst is able to demonstrate to the patient (because the feeling is present in the here and now) that the patient has been, figuratively speaking, hanging the clothes of his father onto the analyst. The patient had not realized how perhaps through his life he has been endowing all "father figures," such as his boss, his teacher, or his commanding officer in the military service, with acting in rejecting and manipulative ways toward him. This misperception, which had previously been unconscious, is now understood by the patient. He can correct his understanding because it is now conscious, and then go on to live and interact in more constructive ways with "father figures." It is as if he learns to live now as an adult, rather than as a child. From the standpoint of ego state therapy we might say that he has removed his ego energies from a child state and invested them into a more adult and contemporary one.

This transference reaction is a powerful psychoanalytic technique, because it involves a reliving of the past, not merely a remembering. It occurs also in ego state therapy (Phillips, 1994; Watkins & Watkins, 1990a). It may be facilitated when the patient is in a hypnotic state, and since hypnosis is a kind of regression, the regression of transference reactions may be precipitated earlier in the treatment (Fromm, Erika, 1968).

Therapists often are somewhat "seduced" by the patient into behaving like the parent of the past. They, too, are influenced by transference reactions. When the therapist unconsciously views the patient as perhaps a younger brother figure, and then talks to or behaves toward that patient like he or she would toward that brother, then the therapist is experiencing "countertransference." The purpose of personal treatment for psychoanalytic therapists is to resolve their own transferences, so that it will not confound the treatment of their patients.

Resonance

Resonance, like transference, is an emotional response between two people, but while in transference the other person is treated as an object, a "not-me," in resonance the other is experienced as part of one's own self.[1] Loving family members often resonate with one another. They coexperience each other's successes, failures, joy, and pain. The optimally functioning "therapeutic self" maintains a balance between objectivity and resonance with one's patient. Too much objectivity and the patient does not feel truly understood. Too much resonance results in therapist and patient coexperiencing a *folie a deux*.

A new patient brought a number of his childhood pictures to his first session of therapy and wanted to show them before he began discussing his case. Some therapists might have failed to notice his badly bruised thumb (with which he held the photos) or have impatiently pressed the patient to get on with the treatment rather than continue what could have been regarded as simply an irrelevant, time-wasting, or resisting activity.

Other therapists, more cognitively oriented, may have made a perfectly normal and sincere intellectual inquiry, such as, "What happened to your thumb?"

However, this particular therapist (HHW) felt the pain he might have suffered. With concern in her voice she made a "resonant" response: "I'm so sorry you hurt your finger."

The patient, who had come from a family in which he had been ignored and neglected, immediately brightened up. He eagerly described the small accident which had injured the thumb. The therapist noticed that from that time on her relationship with the patient was much closer and trusting.

A general principle, perhaps in all therapy, is the following dictum: *Don't do what the parents, or whoever reared the patient early in life, did wrong in the eyes of the patient, whether it is ignoring or abuse.* That statement is particularly true if the patient tests out the therapist to see if abuse is forthcoming sooner or later. For example, a patient who has been sexually abused as a child may act seductively toward the therapist. If the therapist does not understand this behavior as a test but is seduced into action, then not only can the therapist's career be threatened, but also the patient is certainly damaged, sometimes irredeemably so. In this way the therapist has proven to the patient that once again those who seem close are only abusers in disguise. Whether conscious or unconscious, that conclusion is harmful to the patient, to the therapist, and to the relationship.

The perception of abuse lies in the mind of the patient. It cannot be proven or disproven, but its importance should not be overlooked. The word "parents" in the foregoing dictum could be substituted for anyone the patient perceived as being abusive. The patient's perception of abuse is *experientially* true for the patient. Whether consciously remembered or uncovered under hypnosis, that perception needs to be honored. Verifiable truth belongs in a court of law, not in a therapist's office (Watkins, J., 1993a). Healing entails the experiencing and witnessing of what lies in the patient's mind. The world in the past may not have seen any physical or psychological abuse of the child, but that does not mean that the child did not *feel* abused; the opinion of others does not matter.

There are no perfect parents. We are imperfect human beings, even while trying to do better; but more important we have limited control over the perceptions of our children. The child's life experience is limited, its conclusions are naturally narcissistic, and its thinking is concrete and literal.

One patient with a lifelong low-level depression and lowered self-esteem was regressed via an affect bridge technique (Watkins, J., 1971) to the origin of her negative feelings. In the regression she felt herself standing in a crib, listening to mother and father crying in the living room. She heard mother pleading, "I don't want you to go" and father responding, "I don't want to go but I have to." She concluded father was leaving because of her, that she must have done something bad but didn't know what. In actuality he was going off to the Korean War. How would any parent know the child had drawn that conclusion? This innocent example does not whitewash in any way the many incidents of real abuse of children in our culture today.

Paradoxically, the replication of the past (transference) does not exist only in the patient's outside world, but in the inside world as well. Ego states tend to repeat patterns internally which they experienced externally when the patient was a child (Watkins & Watkins, 1990a). For example, an adult who was rejected as a child will sometimes reject her own inner child ego state as an adult, expressing such astounding comments under hypnosis as, "Oh, I don't want anything to do with her; she's a pest." With such an attitude toward one's inner world, healing cannot take place. It behooves the therapist to be alerted to the possibility for such patterns because they are not uncommon.

Mind/Body Connection

Volumes have been written on the relationship between the mind and the body, both for the professional and the layman. For the professional, Selye (1956) published his landmark work on stress. More recently, for the layman, *Healing and the Mind*, a television series documentary (Moyers, 1993), attracted widespread attention. Awareness of the mind/body connection is apparently becoming more widespread. In every bookstore, paperback and hardcover books on stress line the shelves. The contents instruct how to prevent it, what to do about it, how to rid oneself of the causes, etc., in order to feel better emotionally and physically.

Psychosomatic medicine, a very literal reference of the influence of the mind on the body, is not a medical specialty per se but rather the milieu with which every doctor works. Stress is probably a broader term for what used to be called the fight/flight reaction. This reaction is actually part of our mammalian survival mechanism. The mammal, when threatened, either fights (anger) or flees (fear). The animal may also freeze temporarily, like a rabbit in an open field, but then flees. The human being also reacts similarly. However, unlike the animal, it adds one important dimension. It might not express either fear or anger in behavior, or release it in some other way, but rather repress it in the body. Sometimes there is conscious awareness in doing so, sometimes not. Therein lies the problem. In holding on to fear, anger, and other negative emotions in the body, the human being puts him- or herself under physiological stress. A modicum of stress helps us survive. Too much produces wear and tear on the total system.

The animal responds with the fight/flight reaction when the threat is physical. With human beings the threat very often is psychological, but the body responds as if the threat were physical. The anticipation of a difficult college examination may produce heart palpitation, shallow breathing, tight muscles, cold hands and feet—all stress symptoms, even though there is obviously no physical danger.

Stress produces these and other symptoms in the body. They become relevant in ego state therapy when part of the personality (an ego state) is upset for whatever reason. That feeling may manifest itself in some kind of physiological symptom. If that symptom is in the muscles, then a tight chest may produce pain. If in the stomach, an ulcer may be the complaint. There are a myriad of possibilities of stress symptomatology, and these symptoms can be indicators that lead to an ego state that contains the distressed feeling. For example, using a somatic bridge instead of an affect bridge, with or without formal hypnosis, can lead to a significant life event or to an ego state to which the physical discomfort is connected.[2]

The affect bridge (Watkins, J., 1971) is a procedure for tracing the origin of an inappropriate feeling or emotion in the present. In the somatic bridge (Watkins, J., 1992b, p. 62), instead of concentrating on an affect, the patient is asked to focus on the part of the body so affected, and it is suggested that this physical feeling will take the patient back to the original experience. Often the patient will re-experience some trauma of significance that needs to be worked through and mastered.

The somatic bridge can be useful to let the physical symptom, such as a pain or an ulcer, speak for itself. Such a technique might evoke an ego state, or it might not. In any event, no harm is done, and there is some relief in the expression of the feeling. Even without hypnosis it can be useful to say, "Let the throat talk! Let the pain say what it wants to say! Listen to what the stomach wants to tell you!" or whatever seems appropriate.

Sometimes an ego state presents itself very clearly through psychosomatic symptoms. Phillips (1993) devotes a whole article to the treatment of somatic expressions of trauma in ego state therapy. Using hypnotic techniques she demonstrates the utility of using bodily sensations to extricate the patient from trauma. In childhood trauma, abuse usually involves pain to the body in some way. It begets dissociation and the development of ego states. Using stress symptomatology to contact ego states, therefore, can be a subtle but productive inroad for conducting ego state therapy.

The above categories provide understanding for the therapist on how to proceed toward the therapeutic goal desired by both patient and therapist. However, such information is best obtained gradually – not by a shopping list of questions at the first meeting. Interrogation is threatening. Sometimes very little questioning is necessary when the answers are obvious. For example, when a dependent child state appears, the need for a helping ego state is clear.

Attitude Toward Ego States

Upon first meeting with an ego state the therapist's attitude sets the tone for future interaction. Since most ego states were created when the patient was a child, the best way to communicate is to think like a child. That may not be easy for a therapist who has been accustomed (and perhaps specifically trained) to think logically. Listening carefully and with respect is the hallmark of all good therapy.

Resonating with an ego state's feelings will create an ally. Acceptance of its opinions without criticism does not imply agreement or disagreement, but suggests the willingness to understand its position. To assume that "everyone" is listening provides a tactical safeguard. The therapist is less likely to make an error that will infuriate an ego state other than the one being addressed. It is a gross error to express to one ego state that it is more cooperative, nicer, or better in some way than other ego states. And it can be fatal to therapy to suggest that some ego state should be eliminated entirely. These attitudes can significantly increase resistance.

The above attitudes need not imply lack of strength by the therapist. The stamina of fearlessness is an asset in dealing with malevolent states. They have little respect for weakness. However, that strength must be tempered by caring and understanding, otherwise a fight can ensue, which the therapist is bound to lose. And if the therapist loses, so does the patient.

Ego states and the total personality must understand that the resolution of emotional conflict lies within – not outside – the individual. The world at large will not solve one's emotional problems, even though human beings do have a penchant for blaming others for how they feel and wanting others to do the repair work. Patients commonly have this expectation of their therapists. Unfortunately, some therapists are sufficiently narcissistic to be seduced into such disordered thinking. The end result to the patient can only be increased dependency and eventual disappointment because of the therapist's lack of omnipotence. Such a therapist would probably view the patient as difficult and uncooperative. Under these conditions healing will take place with difficulty, if at all.

Since healing must come from within, the therapist should listen carefully to follow the lead of the patient, to understand when intervention is appropriate, and to know when to be silent and let inner forces resolve problems. A useful admonition is to *follow before you lead*. A simple method for following an ego state's conversation without influencing or suggesting is to repeat what the ego state says. It is a subtle way of implying that one hears and is paying attention. It also provides an echo for the patient's own words.

LONELY AND REJECTED CHILD STATES

For example, if an internal child state feels lonely and rejected because of abandonment experiences in childhood, the solution lies in someone nurturing within the system, not by a nurturing adult in the outside world. The depressed patient cannot be cured by marrying someone who is not depressed. The anxiety-ridden person is not relieved of fear because others are not afraid. That concept may be obvious to the clinician, but not necessarily to the patient. Complaints about one's world may be legitimate, but they do not provide the healing of pain that stems from the past, whether or not it is reinforced in the present.

A patient who was abused as a child is likely to view the adult world as uncaring, and perhaps even seek out those who don't care in order to maintain that belief, because once established, beliefs tend to have an autonomy of their own. However, the solution lies in treating the child state that was abused, not in trying to change the patient's external world, even though external changes may be necessary at times. Too many patients lament their present life situation but never change themselves. Some try to get the therapist to solve their problem for them. Some make unrealistic emotional demands. Some expect intercession in the outside world. If the therapist does not set limits and accedes to unreasonable demands (whether explicitly or implicitly made), there is a likelihood of overdependency in the patient. Then effective therapy through constructive inner change stops, and the therapist is regarded simply as a nurturing parent whose purpose is to relieve pain.

The younger the child the more it perceives itself to be the center of its universe. This narcissistic normalcy produces guilt when the child is abused.

It has no awareness of the motivations of others. Its lasting impression, especially if the abuse is repeated, is that it is bad. The conclusion at this biological level can only be: "It's my fault." Therefore, it becomes important for the therapist to convince the child ego state that the abuse was not its fault in order to relieve that underlying guilt and shame—often not a simple process.

The Problem of Dependency

A certain degree of dependency is desirable in a good therapeutic relationship. The patient who trusts and needs the therapist will be positively motivated and constructively oriented. The therapist must be willing to make a commitment to the patient and be willing to accept and tolerate a degree of dependency. If one insists on being too objective, a resentful patient may reject the therapist and terminate treatment, particularly if the patient is dissociated with well-formed, needy child states.

There is a possible dilemma here for the therapist. No dependency or overdependency in the therapeutic relationship may well sabotage the process. J. Watkins (1978a) has described this conflict in considerable detail as a balance between objectivity and resonance. When we are objective we view the patient's problems like an outsider, unaffected by them emotionally. We do not contaminate our perception and understanding of the patient by our own feelings, experiences, or "transferences." When we resonate, we use our whole self through temporarily introjecting the patient and his situation, then change that introject from object to subject (hence egotize it), so that we can coexperience what he or she is going through. This affords a more sensitive and deeper understanding, but with possibilities of personal contamination.

If we are completely objective, we do not become involved enough in the patient's problem and needs. There is inadequate dependence that is permissible. When we resonate too deeply without appropriate, objective safeguards, we encourage overdependency. The secret is to balance the two.

Building Trust

The first and most important task for the therapist, and a "must" before undertaking serious therapeutic work, is to establish trust. Trustworthiness is conveyed by the subtle impact of one's beingness, by nonverbal cues, and by honesty of expression.

Childhood stress and trauma often create feelings of distrust in ego states formed at that time. They expect parent figures (and therapists) to lie to them.

Honesty is generally a good policy in life, but in therapy with dissociated patients, it is crucial. Underlying ego states or alters are waiting for the therapist to slip with a lie. If the therapist says to a patient under hypnosis that he or she loves part of the personality, even a young, helpless child state, that word may imply to the state that the therapist will nurture it forever. That is a lie. Ego states make note of such statements and draw their own child-like conclusions. The therapist cannot be there forever. Even if one could, such behavior would not be healing. One would have a small child on one's hands inside an adult body forever. Nurturing, in order to be permanently healing, must come from within the patient.

One ego state finally trusted me when I (HHW) said I would not abandon her unless the waking personality fired me; only then would I no longer see her. That statement of truth impressed her because the abuser in her life always lied to her. Simply saying, "I will never abandon you" could easily have been interpreted as a lie.

Every behavior, whether verbal or nonverbal, is scanned by the patient, especially by those who experienced abuse as children. The basic question for them is: "Are you to be trusted?" Until they can find at least a tentatively positive answer to that question, therapy will be on hold or proceed very, very slowly.

In order not to prevent gross errors that destroy trust, it is wise to assume that everyone is listening. That situation may not be so, but such an attitude provides a safeguard against antagonizing an ego state unnecessarily. It is understandable that ego states might be angry at the therapist by the very nature of disrupting a system that has been in operation for many years. Few human beings like disruption from whatever is established and therefore predictable. The same is true for ego states. Furthermore, ego states have much at stake to maintain the status quo, even if that system is damaging to psyche or soma. They view the system from a child's point of view, concretely, or at least at the age level of thinking when they came to be. Some ego states may evolve and grow with the patient, such as the ones that say, "I've always been with her." Others, born out of trauma, remain in the trauma, where time stands still. The body matures, the years advance, but the traumatized child remains in the trauma in its thinking and behavior.

When activating an ego state, it needs to be treated with courtesy, even if its thinking seems naive or preposterous to the therapist. An ego state is not a thing or a process. It is a part-person, and as such it wants to be accorded the dignity of being heard with respect.

Resonating with each ego state and treating it as you would want to be treated is akin to following the Golden Rule. There will come a time for confrontation, for breaking down defenses, for making changes in the thinking for the good of the whole system, but first there is the period of acquaintance, understanding, building trust. In that way each state can feel accepted.

In establishing good relationships with each state, the inclusion of seemingly malevolent ones is paramount (Goodman & Peters, 1995; Watkins & Watkins, 1988). Malevolent states are often protective in origin. Originally they were adaptive, at least temporarily. Their internal behavior was maintained and strengthened by continued reinforcements. For example, a malevolent state may view its protective function as being increasingly important if the child's abuse is continued. In working with such a state, it becomes essential to underscore its protective function so that eventually it understands its "benevolent motivation." Then, perhaps, change to more benevolent behavior is possible. Sometimes, in a very fragmented patient, elimination of a state may be necessary, but that needs to be done with caution and with the help of other ego states. The therapist has no magic wand with which to extricate an internal energy system.

One patient at a mental hospital was told to get rid of "Wanda" because "*she* was the problem." The patient objected on the grounds that Wanda was simply a child state who needed help. Furthermore, "What am I supposed to do? Just say poof, go away?" The patient was wiser than her caretakers.

In constructive states, the reinforcing of strengths provides a resource for those who are not as strong or for those who are weak and helpless. For example, the hypnotized patient may be an adult state with understanding and well-meaning. That state can be a resource. Or a nurturing part of the personality can be a source of help to others on the inside. In working with therapists as patients, I (HHW) often find a nurturing part, which represents their therapeutic caring. Lacking that resource within them, they probably would not have been attracted to this profession.

Integration versus Fusion

As repeatedly stated, the goal of ego state therapy is a greater personality integration, whether in severe dissociative patients like multiple personality disorders or in the lesser neurotic conditions and normal behavioral problems.

However, from our point of view, integration and fusion are not synonymous. Fusion suggests an amalgamation of all states into a single unit. It also implies a ceremony produced for such unity. Since we believe that the normal human being is not "fused," as evidenced by the "hidden observer" studies (Hilgard, 1986), our goal is not fusion.

Integration implies cooperation in a mutual needs-meeting resolution of differences. Sometimes two or more ego states find that their needs and the expression of those needs are so similar that it is no longer necessary or advantageous to divide their energies and be separate. They may simply decide to hold hands and stay together. But that is their choice, not the therapist's.

Paradoxically, ego state therapy does not increase dissociation – it decreases it. If an ego state is split off during trauma in childhood, the entity retains the feelings of that experience and the thinking of that moment in time. It does not grow up with the rest of the personality. It is as if that ego state were encased in a prison in which time had frozen and stood still. And the impact of that traumatic experience contains *its* belief of how the world acts in the here and now. As communication between different ego states is facilitated by the therapist, the boundaries separating them become less rigid, more permeable. Information can be shared and dissociation is lessened. Each ego state feels less isolated.

We move now to specific tactics and techniques for implementing these principles of ego state therapy. Most of these (unless specifically stated otherwise) have been developed by HHW. Through therapeutic intervention by various techniques ego states can learn to perceive the world in more realistic ways, and can then constructively interact with other states to become part of a cooperating whole.

9

TECHNIQUES AND TACTICS OF EGO STATE THERAPY

Contacting Ego States

To deal with an ego state one must first contact it, and if the patient is not a true multiple personality, one generally needs to use hypnosis to do so. There are many ways to contact ego states. The most direct way is to hypnotize the patient and ask if there is a part that feels different from the main personality or that feels an emotion the therapist knows is counter to what the patient feels in the waking state. In other words, the purpose is to find out if there is a part of the personality that is in conflict with other parts and that is available under hypnosis. The therapist can add: "If there is such a separate part, then just say, 'I'm here.'" However, the first time this is done, it is important to add a disclaimer, as follows: "But if there is no such separate part, that's just fine," or words to that effect. The purpose is to avoid producing an artifact. It is possible for a very good hypnotic subject to produce whatever he or she thinks the therapist may want. However, an artifact will not usually last or produce meaningful results, because it will not represent a real and already existent component of the personality. Artifacts are not energized by basic needs within the individual and tend to be transitory unless reinforced by the therapist. Probably the worst that can happen is confusion and a waste of treatment time.

Another method of contacting an ego state, after the initial hypnotic induction, is to suggest descending plush-covered stairs together with the therapist. (Counting slowly to twenty, a moderate number, deepens the trance.) The concept of walking down the stairs with the patient reinforces the therapeutic relationship and reassures the patient that he or she is not alone in whatever may ensue. In fact, it is generally good policy to accompany the patient in hypnosis, unless the patient indicates otherwise. In hypnosis the thinking tends to be concrete and literal. Many patients have experienced abandonment in their past and expect such in the present, whether from their immediate world or from their therapist. The therapist's offer to walk downstairs with the patient indicates caring and support.

At the bottom of the stairs, it is worthwhile to suggest a room with a couch and a chair and "other furniture." The imagery is therefore partially structured and partially unstructured, so that both therapist and patient furnish the room with their respective imaginations, setting a scene that is determined in partnership. To continue the fantasy one can say, "As we walk into this room, you sit on the couch while I sit on the chair." The purpose of this positional distinction is to allay any possible apprehension as to what the therapist might be doing. In the concrete thinking of hypnosis such a statement makes clear there is no intention of bodily harm. With a patient who has been physically abused as a child, such a viewpoint is particularly meaningful and possibly relieving. A feeling of safety with the therapist is extremely significant.

In addition to this setting, an oblong table with chairs can be suggested if the therapist anticipates that several ego states might enter the scene. That anticipation will depend upon knowledge obtained from previous sessions. In the logic of concrete thinking oblong tables are more easily expandable if needed. Fraser (1991) published a variation of this table technique.

It is not necessary that the setting be a room. However, a room has an element of containment and therefore privacy and safety. The same room can be used many times. It becomes a familiar place for similar work. An open area may be viewed by the patient as subject to intrusion by the world, past or present, and hence unprotected and dangerous.

If the therapist decides on the use of a table, then the simple statement, "Let's sit at the end of the table" will suffice. At this point the patient may regress into a child state without any suggestion. One patient expressed surprise:

> Oh, I have braids! And a blue and yellow polka-dot dress. And red sandals! I feel 10 years old.

Obviously, an immediate transformation like this has a purpose. Such an ego state has a need and wants to be heard by the therapist. This type of change is much more likely to occur after ego states have already been clearly identified, rather than at the beginning of therapy.

Ego states tend to be cautious and protective. They want to make sure they are safe before exposing themselves. The more they have been abused in the past, the more this statement is likely to be true. Therefore, patients with true MPD (DID) are particularly careful and suspicious of the new therapist. Sometimes it takes a long time before certain alters will appear. They test out the attitude of the therapist behind safe barriers. If the therapist does not believe in the MPD diagnosis, they may never reveal themselves, but still influence the overt personality behind the scenes. That is why ego states/ alters tend not to reveal themselves to skeptical clinicians or researchers, those who already disbelieve in the reality of such dissociation. It is not uncommon to hear skeptics say, "In my years of practice I have never seen a multiple." In all probability they never will.

With the setting in the hallucinated room established, it is time to evoke an ego state if one or more are available at this point in therapy. Speaking to the patient, one might say, "Please watch the door and let me know what you see," and then ask any of the following questions:

Is there someone who might come in who knows about _____?

who wants to be heard?

who is willing to _____?

who feels different from (name of patient)?

Adding, "But if there is no such separate part, that's just fine" will obviate the possibility of artificial cooperation. If the patient reports seeing nothing, a separate ego state may or may not exist. It may mean that one is not suffi-ciently formed to be a separate vocal or visual entity, because the segments of the personality are very permeable. Or, it could be that no one is willing to make an appearance at this time. And it is also possible that the ego state only reveals itself through the body, either kinesthetically or via psychosomatic symptoms.

It is not wise to search for all possible ego states within a given individual. Such a tactic may produce artifacts. Rather, separate out those ego states pertinent to a given problem the patient wishes to resolve. It is very impor-tant that the clinician provides a setting that will permit an already existing ego state to emerge spontaneously without directly suggesting this. An artifi-cial response designed to please the clinician is not the goal of therapy.

Diagnostic Exploration

After the patient has indicated the presence of someone in the hallucinated room, it is time to get acquainted. Without a rigid method of interviewing, both the therapist and the patient may need to learn several things about the ego state.

1. *Age and origin.* "How old was (name of patient) when you came to be?" If a specific age is given then ask, "What was happening at that time?" The specific age gives a clue to a possible trauma that may need to be abreacted at a future session. Sometimes the ego state will simply respond with a clear, "I've always been with her," a statement that does not suggest trauma.

2. *Name.* "What name would you like me to call you?" If it resists a name, "Is it all right if I call you by the age you gave me (e.g., The Eight-Year-Old)?" Since the ego state has appeared, it stands to reason that it wants to be heard. If the therapist expresses interest in the opinions of the ego state, then that state is most likely to agree to a designation that will bring it forth under hypnosis. Persons want to be heard, even part-persons.

3. *Needs.* "What needs do you have?" or more indirectly, "What do you want (name of patient) to do?" The satisfaction of needs are vital in ego state therapy. By satisfying needs, cooperation can be established. Needs are normal, but the internal behavior to achieve those needs can be destructive. Human beings have achievement needs, play needs, dependency needs, protective needs, destructive needs, safety needs, etc. Such emotional necessities are all part of being a social human being.

4. *Function or internal behavior.* The problem arises internally when an ego state has, for example, a strong achievement need and then nags and criticizes other states to achieve a goal that is never good enough. The surface symptom can then be in the form of depression or anxiety. The total personality can never feel good about its achievement. There is always something undone, something not good enough, something that could have been accomplished earlier, etc. The total personality feels ill at ease, dissatisfied, disappointed in itself. An ego state is usually willing to change its internal behavior if its underlying need is being met. Perhaps it can be persuaded to behave differently in order to satisfy that need. However, another ego state must be contacted to help in this needs-meeting process in order to effect conflict resolution. That does not imply this process will be simple. Ego states can be tenacious and disbelieving.

5. *Degree of permeability.* Is the ego state aware of anyone else within that inner world? That is to say, who knows whom, and what are the attitudes toward each other? Obtaining such information gives an expanding picture of the total system.

6. *Gender.* Ego states are not always the same gender as the patient. If a female patient was abused by a male as a child, then at least one ego state is likely to be male. The reason is not related to sexuality per se but to the concept of strength. As one ego state said very clearly, "I have to be male; only males have strength." That ego state represented her introjection of an overpowering abusive male when she was three years old. It was her way of

protecting herself unconsciously, though not in reality. Having introjected an abusive male at the moment of painful trauma, it only understood pain. Its logic was as follows: "I have to hurt her or the world will hurt her more." Thus she suffered from many psychosomatic symptoms any time she came close to males. "He" hurt her to keep men and the world away, ironically a protective function.

Surveying Ego State Interactions

Mapping is a technique used with MPD (DID) clients to understand what alters exist and who relates to whom. The same principle can also be applied to covert ego states but perhaps with lesser complexity. The most intriguing system of mapping the authors have ever seen was shown by a therapist in Canada who had devised a wall hanging of intertwining threads of differing colors. Each thread represented an alter; and when an alter was integrated with another or with a group of alters, the therapist and this complex MPD patient would combine the appropriate threads. This tapestry was a clear, concrete representation of how far the therapy had progressed. Even the audience could determine what was yet to be done, without any knowledge of the details of the case.

Ego state therapy would probably not require such elaborate means of representation, but one still needs to know who is involved in the problem at hand and who knows whom. In other words, relationship between states is pertinent to therapy. Again, just as with the concept of interviewing, rigid interrogation of one ego state after another is not wise. It may remind an abused patient of rigidity experienced in the past. If the therapist has contacted only one ego state, it is simple to ask it, "Are you aware of anyone else in there?" and proceed accordingly.

With one of my (HHW) patients, only a few covert ego states were involved in the therapy, even though her abuse as a child had been so severe that one might have expected an MPD diagnosis. One may wonder why some severely abused children do not grow up to be true multiple personalities. There must be some genetic influence for such differentiation. The three significant parts were the hypnotized patient who was ineffectual, the observer who gave information, and a malevolent one whose fundamental need was to protect but who acted like the abuser. There seemed to be no resource, such as a nurturing part, available. And the protector's rigid thinking and malevolent behavior were certainly not constructive in the present. This case was very complicated and difficult. It is described in more detail in chapter 14.

Sometimes, for whatever reason, an ego state cannot or will not speak directly to the therapist. That may not be a problem. The resolution of conflict lies within the personality and must be carried out by the ones within. Furthermore, it is not the purpose of ego state therapy to increase dissociation by conversing with an ego state for no specific therapeutic purpose. In family therapy the goal is for family members to interact normally. The therapist intervenes with one member only as long as necessary to achieve a certain change. That principle is also true for ego states.

Ego states, like the less permeable alters in MPD (DID), often contain information or feelings about past experiences that are amnestic to the main personality (the person in the waking state). The original purpose of this process was to protect the overt personality from pain. It was an emotional survival mechanism. At the time such separation from consciousness occurred, it was extremely useful; but it became a detriment to adult functioning. That is why the patient is in therapy. The patient wants to understand why he or she has symptoms that seem to be uncontrollable or why there is amnesia about childhood or how to cure the depression or anxiety unrelated to present life experiences or why reactions are all out of proportion to seemingly innocuous stimuli.

In ego state therapy and in MPD therapy, *co-consciousness* (Beahrs, 1982) between states promotes the erosion of amnestic barriers. Such erosion opens the door to differing states understanding each other. It loosens the rigidity of the repression that inhibits the emotions and the recollections of old trauma which an ego state still retains. Co-consciousness also discourages continuation of the child thinking of the past in the absence of current trauma.

For example, if the table technique is used, the therapist can ask for everyone to enter the hypnotic room and sit at the table so that everyone can meet. Not everyone involved in the problem may come, but the scene is an opportunity for internal dialoguing, relating, and understanding. It may give evidence as to who did not come – also informational. As the hypnotized patient describes each ego state that enters, ask where it would like to sit and beside whom. Such a seemingly polite and social question also gives information about relationships and possible future integration or resolution.

Phillips and Frederick (1995) have published a well organized and comprehensive treatment plan. They call it the "Sari" model, an acronym for four stages of treatment: safety and stabilization, accessing trauma, resolving traumatic experiences, and integration.

An Objective Observer

Sometimes a nonemotional part of the personality is available. It has wisdom; it is nonjudgmental; it has information as to the internal landscape; and it can be a great resource for the therapist. Though not emotional, it does care about the preservation of the total system and is therefore beneficial and benevolent. Its inner function is to observe. Some therapists refer to this entity as the inner mind, the higher self, the center, the natural self, the inner self helper (ISH), (Adams, 1987; Allison & Schwarz, 1980; Comstock, 1991), the observer, etc. My (HHW) method is to mention most of these words and then, if such a state exists, let the patient or the ego state choose what designation it prefers.

One way to evoke this state, if available, is to ask the patient to close his or her eyes and say something like the following:

> In each one of us there is an aspect that knows many things that have happened to us. It acts like an observer but has our best interests at heart. Some people call it the observer, or the natural self, or the center, or the inner mind, or whatever. At times that aspect can be contacted through the fingers of the right or left hand. Imagine that the hand is separated at the wrist so that it operates without your conscious help. If that observing aspect is willing to communicate with me right now, then the index finger will rise. If it is not willing to do so now, then the middle finger will rise.

If there is no response at all, then the patient is not sufficiently hypnotized or an observer is not available. However, the patient should not be made to feel there is something wrong or missing or inadequate.

Whether the index or the middle finger moves, either way there is a response. Obviously, this is a double bind, but under the lessened criticality of even light hypnosis, the patient is not aware of that bind. If the middle ("no") finger rises, then acknowledge:

> Thank you for letting me know that you are not ready to communicate with me now. But if at any time in the future you wish to do so, then just signal me with the index finger of the right (or left) hand. I will try to be aware of your signal.

If the index ("yes") finger rises, then continue:

> Thank you for making yourself known. If it is possible for you to speak to me through (patient's name) vocal cords, then just say, "I'm here." If that is not possible, then indicate your response through the middle ("no") finger. Either way is fine with me.

Cheek (1962) first proposed ideomotor signaling with fingers. (See also Rossi & Cheek, 1988.) This technique is described in greater detail in Chapter 14.

Now it is possible to become acquainted with a valuable asset, one that can lead to partnership, such as with a colleague or even a cotherapist. Such an observer state is most likely to tell the therapist what it knows about the inner status quo, warn about dangerous conditions, give advice, or reveal a myriad other bits of information useful to therapy. It is also possible to include another finger for an "I don't know" or "I don't care to answer" response.

The observer can be asked to take the patient to a certain experience, or to an experience of the observer's choice. For example, "Are you able to take her to where she needs to go to undo whatever is necessary?" If the response is positive, whether through finger signals or verbally, then ask, "Are you willing to do that right now?" Both questions are important. Sometimes the observer reveals its ability to take the patient to an important scene, but not at this moment in time.

Furthermore, the observer can be consulted for advice or for an appraisal of the internal scene. After an abreaction the observer might be able to tell the therapist how effective the abreaction was and if it needs to be repeated. Much information is possible from this entity. In addition, an observer can be used as an intermediary to resistance. For example, one patient moved in and out of hypnosis because of fear. I asked the observer to have the patient look at a TV screen to view some past experience. If the patient agreed, the observer took her to the scene to abreact it. If the observer was not sure of some happening, or of who did what, I had the hypnotized patient look more closely at the screen, which helped her to discern more clearly. This particular observer state was overly protective of the patient and learned that she could handle much more than it thought previously. Despite the seeming objectivity of an observer state, it is only a part of the person, and must not be given the authority to take over the therapy, because the therapist has the advantage of being more objective.

Resolving Internal Conflicts

In order to undo original conflicts it is sometimes necessary to return to those experiences via hypnotic regression, so as to achieve an abreaction. The abreaction will hopefully release the feelings that belong to that time, but which are no longer relevant to the present, and help the ego state to learn something new, something constructive. For example, learning by an ego state that it does not need to be afraid of the abuser of the past, that it no longer is a victim, gives the total personality a feeling of power and relief.

Using the hallucinated table, one or more of the ego states can touch each other. Ego states are energy systems, and touch can be very important. After all, the whole body is an electrochemical system, and ego states represent part of that total system. Touch at this level can evoke all kinds of responses, including pleasure, aversion, temperature change, relief, etc., not dissimilar from the outward touch of one person to another.

At the table one ego state can converse with another, silently or out loud, either by the therapist's suggestion or spontaneously. *Internal dialoguing* is the best way to understand the relationship between states or to purposefully develop a relationship between them. For example, if two or more ego states appear to a patient in the hallucinated room, then the therapist can suggest they speak to each other, silently or out loud. Giving the latter two options provides greater control for the patient. If the conversation is silent, the therapist can always inquire what happened.

When initiating internal dialoguing, a useful statement is as follows: "Say what you want to say to (other state)." However, suggesting what one ego state should say to another is akin to directing a play. It does not spring from internal sincerity and is likely to be ineffective. Allowing the ego state to say what it wishes gives credence to what is communicated. Nonetheless, there can also be some detriment in doing so if the expression is totally negative. The therapist should not reinforce destructiveness of one state upon another. With careful interviewing before any internal dialoguing, such a reaction can be prevented. The destructive one can be worked with alone before it heaps more havoc upon the system.

Transitional Objects

Object-relation theorist Winnicott (1965) held that the child's development from a completely narcissistic self-view of the environment to the establishing of objective perspectives and relations with others, such as the mother, could be facilitated by an intermediate interaction with a *transitional object*. Such an object (security blanket, doll, etc.) provides a baby with an external contact which is real, that is, not hallucinated, and one over which it has control. Baker (1981) has pointed out the importance of this intermediate step especially in the therapy of psychotics.

Child ego states can often be contacted and activated when they are provided with a typical transitional object like one they may have possessed when they were first formed. Objects can also be helpful in diminishing fear. A teddy bear is the most likely candidate for such a purpose. Its neutral gender, its cuddly texture, its firmness yet softness, its size—all suggest the feeling of an innocent child. It can represent an internal hurt child that the patient holds in the therapy office, at home, or both. The patient can speak to the bear and give reassurance, or whatever positive messages are pertinent. The bear, of course, represents part of that internal world, though much more indirectly than if the ego state were being addressed personally. There may be less threat in speaking to the object, rather than directly to the ego state. Furthermore, not all ego states are sufficiently separated, so that an overt voice is available. An object also gives distance when emotional distance is necessary. At one time a patient's child state was reluctant to reveal an experience of traumatic nature because of the early threat of reprisal. I had her speak to the bear and tell it that it's okay to reveal the pain during a dream, and "it" did. The entire procedure was within the control of the patient, a much better approach than trying to force an ego state to reveal its contents when not ready to do so.

Abreactive Techniques

No discussion of ego state therapy techniques would be adequate without significant attention to the use of abreactive procedures.[1] Abreactions are an integral part of many different approaches including psychoanalysis (Freud & Breuer, 1953; Reich, 1949), hypnoanalysis (Watkins, J., 1949, 1992b), primal-scream therapy (Janoff, 1970), and certain behavioral therapies, such as flooding or implosive therapy (Stampfl, 1967).

There are many variations, but the essential element is the release of bound emotions through their overt expression, verbally and/or behaviorally. In ego state therapy, abreactions are an extremely powerful technique–which we have employed frequently.

During World War II one of us (Watkins, J., 1949) found that through abreactions many war neuroses (now usually called posttraumatic stress disorder), such as conversion reactions involving hysterically paralyzed hands or legs, phobias, and amnesias, responded favorably to the release (usually under hypnosis) of repressed or dissociated feelings. Grinker and Spiegel (1945) were then conducting abreactions with similar cases but with sodium amytal or sodium pentothal instead of hypnosis.

Abreactions can be performed on an entire patient or on a single ego state once it is activated. For example, an individual reported to me (JGW) that when he was eight years old his mother, whom he loved greatly, had died, and he had been told what a brave little man he was for not crying. I suspected immediately that there must be an eight-year-old child state filled with repressed grief. The child state was activated through hypnotic regression and induced to give full vent to the repressed or dissociated anguish, thus relieving a continuing source of depression and other symptoms.

However, it may not be sufficient to abreact the feelings of only one ego state, especially in the more rigid structure of the MPD (DID) patient. Since the main personality repressed those feelings into that alter or ego state in the first place, it must eventually take back those feelings and express them. In that way integration is feasible.

The essential elements of an abreaction are as follows:

1. Abreactions are best accomplished through the reliving of a traumatic experience that the patient could not completely face at the time.

2. Through the ego-strengthening of a strong relationship with the therapist, the patient (probably now much older) is enabled to confront the original traumatic situation, re-experience it, release the bound affect, and achieve cognitive meaning.

3. In the case of child abuse this procedure may mean confronting the *introjected representation* of the abuser, mastering it, and recovering the self-power lost at the time of the original situation (Watkins & Watkins, 1978). If the patient is afraid I (HHW) sometimes say, "You are not alone now. There is not only the child state, but also the adult energy; and if you wish to use my energy in addition, then I will touch you on the shoulder if that's okay with you." (I always ask permission to touch.) Such allying gives the patient courage to face the terrors of the past.

Patients who have recalled child abuse in therapy have sometimes attempted to rectify this by directly accusing parental abusers or suing them in court. Such outside confrontation may not change the internal system, which is the function of therapy. Therapeutic resolution must come within, since the malevolent object representation of the abuser, internalized at the time, and not the old person of the present, is usually the source of current dissociation, neurotic conflict, and torment. Justified or not, suing in court is revenge.

Recently, patients who have confronted parents on the basis of recollections of abuse derived in therapy have themselves (as have their therapists) been accused and sued for "false memories." The problem should be resolved *within the treatment*, and therapists should not try to be legal counselors. The pros and cons of revenge need to be discussed at the waking level.[2]

Since the affect was repressed or dissociated because the patient could not face and master the traumatic situation, those patients whose adjustment borders on psychosis should be abreacted only with great care. If the combined ego strength of the patient, plus that loaned by the therapist, is not sufficient to cope with the severity of the trauma, then the patient is retraumatized. No mastery experience takes place. When in doubt, work on the relationship.[3]

4. If the conditions for an abreaction seem propitious, then the decision

may be to proceed. This generally means to go in thoroughly, continue until the bound affect has been completely released, and understanding plus mastery is achieved. In other words, either complete or don't do the abreaction. The worst of all is a half-done abreaction, which has breached the patient's defenses, opened him or her up and then left him that way, because either the patient and/or the therapist "could not take it," for example, facing the violent expression of emotions—fear, hate, grief, etc. A properly done abreaction must end with some closure. Some therapists may find they are not personally prepared to involve themselves in these strong, emotional experiences. Such practitioners would be wise to think twice before conducting abreactions.

5. The patient is hypnotically regressed to the moment of the trauma and the experience is vivified.

6. Through encouragement and coexperiencing, the patient is induced to relive the traumatic event over and over. Shouting, screaming, cursing, pounding are all encouraged. "Say or do whatever you want" or "Tell him he can never again do that to you," etc., when the bound affect is rage. Or "You're frightened. It's really scary. You'd like to get away," etc., if the emotion to be released is fear. If a patient says to me (HHW), "I'm afraid he'll get me later on," I simply say, "I won't let him!"

7. When the emotion is exhausted, when the patient is physiologically and psychologically exhausted (as evidenced by a fading away of the violent expressions), *then, and not before,* comes the time for reassurance and reinterpretations. The abused child, for example, needs to learn that the abuse was not her fault.

8. Abreactions involve the principle of counter-conditioning or systematic desensitization as studied by learning psychologists in the laboratory (Wolpe, 1982). They may need to be repeated, perhaps immediately after the first time and during the same session, perhaps again the next day, the next week, etc., until the patient no longer shows the symptoms that resulted from the original situation. Each repetition of the traumatic situation is usually experienced less violently until true extinction has been reached. The event then becomes a matter of simple memory, not relived pain.

A battalion surgeon was referred to me (JGW) because of a hysterical tremor in his right hand. He complained of the humiliations he had suffered at the hands of a commanding officer and vividly threatened what he would do if, "I could get that man on my operating table." The operating table was hallucinated under hypnosis. The patient, screaming, repeatedly "stabbed" the hallucinated abuser, with the therapist shouting encouragement. ("Give it to him. It's what he deserves," etc.). After two fifteen-minute abreactions he emerged from trance, and with a feeling of triumph, held up his right hand. The tremor was gone. Transference interpretations could then be accepted, related to how the commanding officer had precipitated unconscious memories of abuse from a dominating father.[4]

In the case of patients who suffer quite severe pathology, such as multiple personality disorder (dissociative identity disorder) it may be necessary to run attenuated or "slow burn" abreactive releases (Kluft, 1988). The patient is told to experience the affect only to the degree to which he is prepared "at this time" to do so, and that the rest will become available later when he is ready.

The Affect Bridge

In the Affect Bridge technique (Watkins, J., 1971), a current feeling may provide the bridge by which one can move from a current situation to an earlier one involving the same feeling.

A young man felt considerable anxiety when confronting an employment manager. He was hypnotized, regressed to the interview, and his fear vivified. Then he was given the following suggestions:

> Your fear is very strong. Everything else is fading. You are forgetting about the office and the employment manager. All you can experience is fear, fear, fear. You are now traveling back in time, like on a railroad, where the track is just fear. You are going back to a time where you first felt that fear. Where are you? What is happening?

The patient then described a scene in which he was a ten-year-old boy standing in front of his father. He had just broken the living room window with a baseball and his father was very angry and going to spank him.

Through the common affect of the fear of an authority figure, he was transferred back to an early experience where that apprehension first originated. By going back and forth between the present employment interview and the confrontation with the angry father he learned why he was afraid when applying for the job. He recognized that the employment manager reminded him of his father. He allocated the anxiety to its proper place in his life, and ceases to be afraid of employment managers.

The above experience is simply a transference interpretation, such as is often the significant moment in psychoanalysis.

In summary, here is the technique: Have the patient experience the affect that is deemed inappropriate at the present time. The affect may already be evident when the patient enters the therapy hour or it may need to be recovered as in the above example. In any event, hypnotize the patient and say, "This feeling will take you back to the very first time you had that feeling; when you arrive there, let me know where you are." The purpose of this statement is to access the sensitizing experience that began the process. There would be later experiences that reinforced the affect, but they would not be as important as the initial one. That initial experience can then be abreacted and the affect altered.

The Somatic Bridge

As mentioned in a previous chapter, the somatic bridge is similar to the affect bridge, except the bridge now refers to a feeling in the body that is possibly related to stress. For example, if the patient is troubled with a tight chest (a very common stress symptom) then, with the patient in the trance state, say, "Concentrate on that tightness; focus on it. Now that feeling will take you back to the first time you had that feeling; when you arrive there, let me know where you are." If the patient arrives at some experience, then the present has been linked to the past. An abreaction may be appropriate.

The Silent Abreaction

Helen Watkins (1980a) developed an abreactive technique that does not require the patient to engage in violent shouting or screaming (such as might endanger the lease on one's professional office).

She pictures for the hypnotized patient a tranquil scene in which she and the patient are walking together on a path in the forest, and which is safe from any intruder. A large boulder blocks the way, which is labeled as the patient's source of frustration. A nonbreakable, thick, stout stick is conveniently nearby, and the patient is urged to pick it up and strike the boulder. The therapist encourages with, "Hit it again. Hit it again. This thing has been in your way all your life. You can move it. You can break it up. You can do anything you want with it. Just keep on going until you are too tired to go on, then signal me again," etc. The whole experience is in imagery, and the patient makes no sound, but finger signals are established so that the therapist knows the patient is following the visualization.

After the exhaustion of this "hitting" phase a pleasant relaxation on a meadow is pictured and pleasurable sensations are suggested. A request is made: "Before we can go to the next step of what we are doing today, I need something from you. What I need is your willingness to say something positive about yourself." For a patient who has been inhibited from expressing anger, accommodating such a request may not be easy. However, since the patient is curious about the possibility of a further pleasant experience, a response is usually forthcoming. Then good feelings are described that spread through the patient's body, first emanating from the patient's new-found hope, and then followed by more pleasure, which is represented as coming from the therapist's belief and confidence in the patient. The relationship is used here to the utmost.

In other words the patient is given a positive reinforcement for the expression of anger against an object that can *symbolize* an abuser, or whatever the patient decides it to be. Typically, in the past the patient has not been permitted to express anger without punishment or other dire consequences. Receiving positive reinforcement now for the release of rage counteracts that earlier learning.

We have no objective studies indicating whether the silent abreaction is as effective as a full-blown release, but it can be administered in greater comfort, and may be the precursor of a more strenuous emotional release. Furthermore, it can be used as psychological homework, simply using imagery.

Brief Ego State Treatment

Ego state therapy can take many sessions but it also can be extremely short. During the second session one patient told me that from previous therapy she was aware of another part of her that she called "Ramblin' Rose." She stated that Ramblin' wanted her to leave the university and return home because she did not belong in this middle class environment. Prior to entering college the patient had been successfully employed as a bouncer in a biker's bar in a small town. She also reported that Ramblin' came out only after two shots of whiskey. (The patient was not an alcoholic.) "Then I could do anything–even dance on the tables." (At 230 pounds that must have been quite a sight!) I hypnotized her and asked for Ramblin'. After a gruff response of "What do you want?" she began to tell me of her history with the patient and how she had protected her since early childhood. I countered with a simple "Then you must love her." That statement threatened her "Hard-Hearted-Hannah" defensive system. She refused to talk to me any more.

At the following appointment, the patient declared, "You're ruining me. I went to a bar this weekend, drank two shots, and Ramblin' didn't come out!" Under hypnosis Ramblin' said, "Oh, don't worry; I was there in case she needed me. But I thought about what you said, and I decided she's got to learn to be responsible for her own behavior." Here was an ideal situation–a protective state in the background while I helped the waking state to adapt to university life. There was no need to continue talking to Ramblin'. (After all, it is not the purpose of ego state therapy to increase or continue dissociation. The purpose is to guide the patient toward healing, conflict resolution, and integration.) Several sessions later I did contact Ramblin' to find out how she fared. She said she was resting and watching, agreed with me that the main personality was growing up, and complimented me on helping her to adjust. Apparently her strong, fearless energy was being incorporated into the waking state, and that is exactly what needed to occur. However, most ego state cases are not so simple to treat or so cooperative, and they can require many more sessions.

Summary

Various techniques, limited only by the therapist's creativity and sensitivity, can be applied together or separately. If sufficiently in balanced resonance with the patient, the therapist will make many less errors than if he or she sees the patient only objectively. The therapist needs to ponder where the resources are within the patient, which ego states need to be helped, and what needs to change in order to achieve therapeutic closure. Ego state therapy can be a complex but satisfying challenge.

Behavior therapists generally believe that true and lasting change requires objective alterations of observable behavior, which have been caused by specific learned, destructive contingencies. Cognitive therapists and some psychoanalysts require that there be a changed verbalized alteration based on a new interpretation of real experiences, either in the present or in the past. These practitioners may see ego state therapy as working greatly with fantasies, imagination, and other covert processes—which it does. However, we should realize that what happens to us, although it may be caused by an original stimulus, is not as important as *how we interpret that experience, what it means to us.*

The inner, subjective meanings we have may have been caused by actually experienced traumas or other true events. However, the individual who as a child interpreted a mild rejecting behavior on the part of a parent as, "She hates me and abuses me," may construct a malevolent object representation that continually "beats" on the patient, resulting in a lifelong depression. Yet the source of the pain is subjective and based on the child's interpretative and concrete meaning—fantasy or imagination if you will. Cognitive therapists recognize this misinterpretation and seek to change the patient's meaning of the event. However, if their interpretation is only to the conscious individual, and does not reach more covert and infantile states (possible with hypnosis), then there may be no change in the unconscious, malevolent representation. The patient continues to suffer.

We may need to lift repressions, discover true events, and confront them. However, in the last analysis it is the patient's *meaning*, whether having been impacted by an actual, real, noxious event, or the imagined or fantasied interpretation of a possible such event. And it is that meaning which requires changing. That is why so often (as will be seen by the case examples cited) in ego state therapy we may not always be dealing with reality, but often with fantasy. Fantasy representations can create lifelong symptoms as well as reality experiences. It is the acquiring of a harmonious functioning of the inner system that we seek, regardless of its "cause."

10

SPECIALIZED PROCEDURES

Problems of Child States

States introjected in childhood and those resulting from childhood trauma are child states. As mentioned earlier, to be able to think like a child is an asset for the therapist. That statement is valid whether dealing with destructive or with fearful states. For example, one patient told me that there were some states behind the door of the hallucinated room who were afraid of me. I suggested that they could peek in from the doorway, watch and hear me while I spoke to the hypnotized patient, and then decide if I was to be feared. In that way they could gradually become accustomed to me. Isn't that what young children do naturally with strangers? Another time a regressed patient was afraid of monsters coming into her room (Watkins & Johnson, 1982). I told her I had a secret, that I knew how to get rid of monsters, and "Would you like to know my secret?" That is an irresistible question to a small child. Of course, she agreed. I continued, sitting close beside her in order to lend support, and both of us facing an actual door: "Now you watch the door, and as soon as you see a monster come in, say 'Go 'way!' real loud, and the monster will go away," which she did. Not surprisingly, she reported the monster was gone. For a little one, even if in a big body, such a technique is ego strengthening, because it gives the child power and is also age-appropriate. If I had spoken to her adult self, nothing would have happened, and it would not have been helpful in allaying her fear.

Dealing with Fear

Fearful states clearly need help. That can be accomplished by finding a constructive state to care for them, to play with them, or to satisfy whatever need is apparent. Such a needs-meeting process, in order to be effective, must be with the consent of both parties. They need to work out the details of their "contract" with each other through internal dialoguing.

THE SAFE ROOM TECHNIQUE

Using a safe room technique (Watkins, J., 1992b) is another way to make fearful states more secure. The following is an example under hypnosis, using stairs for deepening:

> Now that we are at the bottom of the stairs, let's walk down the hallway. At the end of the hallway is a door to a room of your own choosing, in which you will feel safe and comfortable. As we come closer to the door, look at it carefully and describe the door for me, even the doorknob.

The purpose of the description is to check on what the patient is viewing and also to further focus and thus perhaps deepen the trance. Unless the door is clearly a fantasy one, ask if the door is familiar in order to explore any association that might be meaningful.

> Now I want to ask you a question. Whatever your answer, it's fine with me. Would you like me to come in with you or stay outside the room?

The answer is an index of dependency on the therapist. If the patient indicates "yes," then the therapist opens the door. If "no," then the patient opens the door while the therapist waits outside. Proceed as follows:

> Look around this room of your own choosing in which you will feel safe and comfortable. Find a place where you can sit or lie comfortably. [Pause] Now I'd like you to search for something. What I'd like you to search for is your inner core of strength. That inner core of strength will take symbolic form. It may be part of the animal kingdom, the vegetable kingdom, or the mineral kingdom. If it is part of the animal kingdom, then it could be an animal or human form; if part of the vegetable kingdom, it could be a flower or plant or tree; and if part of the mineral kingdom, it could be an object or maybe even an energy. I don't know what symbolic form it will take. All I know is that inner core of strength exists within you. [Wait for a response and then continue.] Touch that [symbol mentioned], feel it, smell it, know it is part of you. Know it is your friend and will help to strengthen you. [Let the patient comment on the symbol.] This is a place to which you can return any time you wish by just closing your eyes, and walking into this room. No one else is allowed to enter here unless you specifically invite them and only if they say positive things to you. [Arousal.]

The patient's perception of this inner core of strength is very informative. There is a vast difference between a delicate kitten versus a huge grizzly bear, or a lush plant versus a weathered stunted tree. The symbol has its own meaning to the patient and needs to be explored, both under hypnosis and after arousal. As therapy progresses, these symbols may change to reflect the therapeutic progress, or lack of it.

The safe room can be used for a specific ego state or for the total personality, whatever seems appropriate to do. It is a technique that can be practiced at home. The therapist can also put a customized or generalized version on tape for the patient to play at home (Watkins, H., 1990a). Because of the "inner core of strength" suggestion, it serves as both a haven of safety to reduce fear and an ego-strengthening technique.

At one time a patient of mine was afraid at the door of the safe room because the "bad one is here." I said, "Don't worry. I'll hold on to him while you run into the safe room." That maneuver worked fine. By that time I had developed enough relationship for her to believe me. After all, criticality is truly subdued in hypnosis.

In order to prolong the influence of a therapy hour, it may be useful for the therapist to make a personal tape for a specific client, or perhaps a more generic type of tape useful for differing clients. Such a tape, published by HHW (Watkins, H., 1990a) is entitled "Raising Self-Esteem." It promotes the concept of ego states in a tangential way by simply referring to "parts of you" within the context of ego-strengthening suggestions.

THE SAFETY COCOON

An alternative approach for dealing with fear is a fantasied cocoon. Speaking slowly, with the patient relaxed, proceed as follows:

> I'd like you to close your eyes and imagine a font of golden white energy springing from the top of your head, moving down your body, around each arm, and around each leg, so that you are completely surrounded by this imaginary cocoon of energy that lets you move about freely, is invisible to anyone else, but is strong and protects you. It protects you from hurt, from negative words someone might throw at you. If someone throws hurting words at you, it will seem like arrows coming at you, but those arrows hit the cocoon and fall off. Or maybe they stick a little, but they can't get inside. You are in control of that cocoon. If you want to take it off at night, you can, or at any other time you feel you don't need it. Let's try it out. [Then rehearse a problem scene.]

Again it is important to have sufficient relationship built so that the technique will be effective. In order to make sure the patient is following the imagery, it makes sense to check with finger signals or orally that he or she is experiencing what is being described. This technique lends itself easily to interaction with the outside world. That is to say, the patient can carry "the cocoon" around and provide emotional protection when needed. In fact, both the safety cocoon and safe room techniques can be used with the same patient; one does not preclude the other.

These methods are temporary devices. Eventually the fear needs to be ameliorated by the inside system in order to have permanent resolution.

The Ideal Self

This technique, although ego strengthening, lends itself to future progression within the hope of the present. It can be used for the total personality or for one or more ego states. One patient decided to experience the imagery with her whole internal family around her.

Relax the patient and, walking together, describe a pleasant country road with quiet, lovely scenery. With a female patient, for example, proceed with the following or similar wording:

> As we walk along you will notice another path that meets our road up ahead. As you look over to that path you will notice someone walking on that path, someone who looks something like you. Curious, you keep watching that person, who is now entering our road up ahead. You notice that she is wearing what you are wearing today [describe] and with the same hair color and hair style. You notice that this person is walking with confidence, as if she knows where she is going and how to get there. You are intrigued, and you decide to leave me behind to catch up with her. You walk faster and soon you find yourself in step with her, so that when she puts her right foot forward, so do you, and then her left foot and then yours. Now you decide to meld with her, so that her head becomes yours, her body becomes yours, and all those confident feelings that she has belong to you.[1] You stride forward into the future feeling strong and confident.

The above wording needs to be appropriate, of course, to the circumstances of the patient, and how she would characterize her ideal self.

Deceased Targets

In order for a child state to vent anger or grief it is not necessary for the target person to be alive. Anger can be vented at a dead parent or sibling or at whomever the significant abuser was. Sometimes ego states view the deceased as alive in the regressed past. Sometimes they view the deceased as a spirit at whom they can express their feelings. Those feelings can be negative or positive or both. One patient recalled that at age three her beloved grandmother and constant companion died suddenly while baby-sitting the little girl. She thought her grandmother had fallen asleep. When her parents came home, they blamed her for not alerting the neighbors and possibly saving the grandmother's life. She felt terribly guilty. I explained that although her grandmother died so many years ago, grandmother still lived inside of her (the introjection of a significant other) and could still talk with her and be her companion. Under hypnosis she rejoined her wonderful caretaker, who promised she would always be there for her whenever needed.

Another patient entered therapy because of uncontrollable bouts of compulsive crying. He had experienced a devastating emotional blow when his young granddaughter died of leukemia within two weeks of onset. He described how this baby had become the love of his life, how he would play with her and talk to her every day, feeling that somehow she understood. To him there was almost a spiritual quality to the relationship. Aware of his unhappy life, I wondered if perhaps this was the only human being who ever loved him unconditionally and whom he loved the same way in return. He broke into deep sobbing. I hypnotized him, took him into the hallucinated room, and asked him if he could bring "the spirit" of this child into our room. He visualized and dialogued with it.[2] He reported "the little girl" smiled at him and told him her purpose was to teach him the meaning of love, in both receiving and giving. "It was time for me to go, but I will always be with you." After one last bout of crying, he emerged from the session totally exhausted but happy, and the compulsive crying ceased.

Adult States as Helpers

Another method of helping a child state might be for the adult to snatch the child away from an abuser. For example, suppose in the hypnotic fantasy one uses a different scene at the bottom of the stairs, because the therapist decided at this point in the therapy that the hypnotized patient needed *to view* what happened to her as a child, *instead of re-experiencing it*. One can describe a room with a one-way vision screen where what is happening on the other side can be seen. Then the therapist may suggest a consciously recalled setting from childhood, such as the patient as a little girl in her bedroom. "I think someone is coming into the room. Let me know what happens." If what she sees is an abuse scene, the therapist might tell her, "You know you don't have to put up with this any more. You can go over there and rescue her." She may be able to penetrate the one-way mirror or search for a side door and finally reach the victim. Or she may not find the abused child at all. In any event she is motivated to help her (a good therapeutic sign), but other steps may need to be taken before this is possible.

In a scene with another patient, the hypnotized adult and I were standing before a crib with an unhappy baby inside. We discussed whether I should take the baby out of the crib or if it would be better for her to do so. We both agreed *she* needed to do this. She explained very logically, "If *I* do this, *I* can take her to a safe place, and *I* can keep her there."

The Use of Volunteers

When the presence of ego states has already been established, a volunteer state can sometimes be useful to help out a child state.

> Susie, would you look at the door of our room? I'm going to ask a volunteer to come in to help you out. It will be someone who *wants* to do this. I don't know who that might be. Let me know who comes in.

I never use this technique unless I am certain there is a nurturing aspect to the patient. Otherwise I would be reinforcing the negative if no helper were available. (Clients that are therapists themselves almost certainly have a "helping" state somewhere within.) If I know that a helping agent is in the patient, but he or she says, "Nobody's coming," then I say, "You must *want* someone to come." That works well. Many child states who have been abused do not believe they deserve to be helped, because of derogatory messages the patient received as a child. After the frightened one sees someone, I ask for a description. Then we proceed with internal dialoguing and communication with me. The purpose is to meet the child's needs with the agreement of the volunteer.

THERAPIST AS TEMPORARY RESCUER

There have been times that no one else is present except a frightened child state and myself. Under those circumstance I might take her away myself "to a (fantasied) place for safekeeping" until I can find other resources inside the personality. She is in my temporary custody only, somewhat like a child in a foster home waiting for placement. The *internal* family placement, however, is hopefully much more secure and predictable than an "outside" transitional foster home.

The concrete thinking of child states is constantly apparent when trying to help them. This was most clearly depicted when I was conducting a sort of psychodrama (Moreno, 1946), made inwardly "experiential" through hypnosis. One patient's two-year-old ego state wanted to kill her mother with a knife she held, but she was afraid. So she asked me to hold the knife, to which I agreed. Then she turned to her mother and thoroughly expressed rage and anger at her, after which they dialogued and then reconciled. In this scene I was very much of a bystander. I really wasn't needed except to provide silent support.

Ego State "Pain"

Under hypnosis, physical or emotional pain within an ego state can also be drained into an adult state who agrees to accept it. It is essential that *both* agree to the arrangement, since it may have been dissociated into that ego state by the adult state in the first place (see Watkins & Watkins, 1990b). Although it may sound strange, some ego states are reluctant to let go of the pain for fear they might disappear, die, have no power, or have no reason to exist. As one said, "My pain is me!"

On the other hand, if the adult state has repressed the pain for so many years, it also may be reluctant to take it back. Therein can lie a therapeutic problem of significant proportion. In the art of therapy each state needs to be gently persuaded along the lines of its individual logic and ways of thinking, so that it will believe in the advantages of such a change. In the case of one patient, the two contending states finally agreed to a solution. The adult would hold the hurting child in safety and love. Subsequently they were content to stay together, and the result was integration.

An adult state can also contact ego states of various ages (an approach appropriate near the end of therapy) and take on the feelings of each. Or the adult might present a young state with the following explanation: "Your pain is from the past, but I am from your future, and I can handle your pain." With one patient, while the child state "sat on the adult's lap," the adult released the pain out loud, the child felt freed, and the patient experienced a new sense of integration.

Critical States

In coping with critical states, the approach of choice is more likely to be confrontive, logical, or practical. Often a demanding state can be motivated to change if it really understands that an alteration of internal behavior is to its advantage. For example, an ego state whose need is achievement might be willing to change its nagging behavior if it can be convinced that speaking more positively, more supportively, more encouragingly to the one who is procrastinating will bring about more achievement. Sometimes it is useful to suggest trying out this kind of tactic for a few days, allowing the critical one to determine how successful the change was. Then it has the choice of continuing the new behavior or returning to old familiar patterns. Under these circumstance it is wise also for the therapist to contact the state who is procrastinating so as to gain its cooperation and change its behavior. Such a resisting ego state probably needs approval from the critical one. Giving a critical state choice to try something new has great appeal, because such a state often has a need for power and control. To make demands of critical states only sets up conflict with the therapist, a contest that is not won by either therapist or patient. The following is an example of such an interaction that required only one session to be resolved:

The patient felt uncomfortable because she had taken time off from work when she was not sick. In a relaxed state and with eyes closed, I had her image the part that might object to her taking the morning off. She saw herself with her mouth tight and serious. I had her listen to what that self said: "You shouldn't do that!" I asked the patient to find out what the needs were of the part she just heard. She reported that "Should" wants her to work hard to be successful and not play around. "Should's" internal behavior consisted of nagging and making her feel guilty. The results were not satisfying to "Should." I talked to "Should" directly and suggested a change of tactics, that is, to support her, give positive messages, and have faith in her. The voice said, "I tried that last month but she played with her boyfriend all the time." Then I asked "Should" to visualize the one who wants to play. She saw a ten-year-old in a pinafore. "Oh, she looks ridiculous in that dress!" declared "Should." I cautioned "Should" not to be disparaging if she wanted cooperation. I asked the ten-year-old how she felt. "I just decided to get dressed up and play. If she would let me out more often, I wouldn't get so crazy." It was time for compromise. The hypnotized patient entered the scene and worked out a compromise. This process also gave the patient a tool that she could use with self-hypnosis in the future.

The critical, ambitious ego state versus the internal procrastinator may represent an original conflict from the patient's past. For example, a parent long ago may have nagged a youngster to study. Unless the student was happy to do the homework, resistance developed within the child, regardless of the actual behavior of the youngster at that time. With repeated naggings the child introjects this drama and grows up feeling both the "should" side of itself and the "I don't want to" facet of the personality when challenged to achieve.

The Door of Forgiveness

This technique (Watkins, H., 1990c) may or may not involve ego states. Ego states may become obvious as the therapy evolves, but there is no specific attempt to call upon any ego state.

The purpose of the technique is to obviate guilt. When feelings of guilt are the primary symptoms, and the need to relieve that guilt is necessary for healing, then this technique lends itself to that goal.

After the patient is hypnotized and deepened with stairs, proceed as follows:

> We are now at the bottom of the stairs. In front of us is a hallway, at the end of which is the Door of Forgiveness. But before you can enter the Door of Forgiveness, you may need to enter other doors on either side of the hallway. Look down that hallway and note if you can see any doors. [Wait for a response. If the patient specifies viewed doors, then proceed.] Which door would you like to enter first? [Perhaps the patient indicates the first door on the right.] Fine. Let's walk up to that door. Describe the door to me, even the doorknob [Purpose is focusing and familiarity]. Have you ever seen this door before? [Explore.] As we stand here together, I'd like you to open that door and tell me what you see. [Wait for a response.] Let's walk inside.

Now the therapy begins. The patient has gone to a scene that needs to be resolved before he or she can enter the Door of Forgiveness, otherwise what would be the purpose of perceiving a door at all? Now is the time for the therapist to follow, to repeat the patient's sentences, that is, to be very nondirective. The scene will evolve in the way the patient needs to face it. The patient may remain an adult or regress to childhood. It may require an abreaction or simply a new way of perceiving some experience. Ego states might become predominant. One never knows what the content might be. It is clear, however, that something must be resolved that is connected with guilt before the patient leaves the room and shuts the door. The shutting of the door is a way of symbolically leaving something behind, closed off only as a memory.

Resistance is clear when a patient sees only an empty room. It is simple to say, "Well, let's walk in; maybe there's another room." It is not surprising that the patient may not want to face feelings of guilt. However, the very we-ness of the therapist accompanying the patient helps to muster courage.

The structure of this technique lends itself easily to the 50-minute hour, because not all doors need to be finished during one session. With one door completed, the next one can be addressed during the following session.

When all doors have been entered and completed, it is time for the Door of Forgiveness:

> Now let's walk to the end of the hallway to the Door of Forgiveness. As we stand in front of this door, what do you see? [Wait for a response.] Let's open the door. I will stand by the door while you enter this place and experience whatever you need to experience. You can do this silently or out loud. Just let me know when you are finished. [Then arousal from hypnosis.]

This experience can be very poignant—religious, spiritual, or mystical. It is always meaningful, and therefore important for healing.

However, not all patients follow this procedure according to plan. One patient in his thirties had a compulsion to drive his car into any oncoming truck. Very consciously and deliberately he had to hang on to the wheel to prevent an accident. At the onset he had seen a psychiatrist three years before for therapy and medication. Nothing helped. Nothing in his history gave a clue to such self-destructive motivation. I concluded guilt must be the culprit and decided on the Door of Forgiveness technique. At first we passed through two doors involving minor school-time miscreant behavior. At the third door I asked, "What do you see?

"Jesus Christ!" he said in astonishment. "What's He doing here?"

"I don't know," I replied, "ask Him!" A period of silence ensued.

"Jesus said, 'You have desecrated my house and you never paid the price.'"

"What does that mean?"

"Oh, I think I know what that's all about."

I aroused him from hypnosis. He explained that a few years earlier he had come back from Vietnam, angry at God, and had tried to burn his church down. The police did not press charges, and the insurance company of the church paid the $500 damage. Obviously, he never paid the price. In this instance the price had to be paid literally. We set up a payment plan of $10 a month anonymously to the church until the $500 was paid off, and the symptom went away. One never knows what surprising events can occur in hypnotherapy.

The Nonhypnotic Chair Technique

I (HHW) developed this technique for two reasons. It is useful for working out conflicts with patients who have mixed feelings about a problem area and where hypnosis is not appropriate for whatever reason. Also, it is a useful tool to demonstrate in our workshops the evidence of differing feeling states, their influence upon each other, and how the conflict can be resolved.

In our workshop the procedure begins with five movable chairs in a circle, simply for convenience. That many chairs may not be needed. In one's office other objects may be used for sitting, but they need to be movable for the process to work smoothly. After a simple explanation of the need to separate out mixed feelings on the subject, the client sits on one of the chairs, while the therapist sits beside him or her with notepad in hand.

> Larry [for example], you told me you have mixed feelings about _____.
> On the top of this page I'm going to write "Attitude toward _____."
> What I'd like you to do in this chair is to say how you feel about this subject, while I simply record like a secretary on my notepad. Okay? Start out with "I feel" and continue.

The therapist writes on the notepad without interpersonal communication, without eye contact with the client, and without interruption by a slow-writing therapist if at all possible. When the client has expressed one feeling on the topic, the two move to the next chair.

> Now could you find a feeling state that feels differently from chair #1 and express that feeling in this chair?

It is important that the therapist never sits on a chair that has already been used by a feeling state. It destroys the integrity of the therapy. Concrete thinking comes into play, and the patient will not appreciate such lack of regard for that feeling state. The changing of chairs then continues until the client can find no more feelings that are different from the ones already expressed. So far we have dealt with a *subjective* event. Now we turn to what is *object*.

> Larry, would you stand beside me now while I read off to you what chair #1 said. Then just give me a brief description of what chair #1 is like. [Using the neutral word "chair" gives no presupposition of gender.]

Read off the transcript with a resonant voice appropriate to the feeling the client expressed.

Do not allow negative labeling, for example, "He's an idiot." Nudge with a question such as, "Well, what does this state feel?" The therapist writes the description below the transcript on the notepad, in full view of the patient.

> Now, would you give me a name or a title that fits chair #1—a title might be a word you already gave me, like "The Depressed One," or an

actual name. [Record answer on the top of the notepad.] Does he seem older, younger, or contemporary to you? [Record this information under the name.]

If the response is either older or younger, then ask, "Any particular age? Anything come to mind about that age?" Record any bit of relevant data under the age, again in full view of the client. He has constructed a form with content, a structure that has meaning to him, and thus comes to life. As each chair description is thus completed, tear off the page and place it on the appropriate chair. When this process is complete, read off a summary of the transcript, the description, the name or title and age of each chair. For example,

Chair #1 said _____, you described it as _____, named it _____, and it felt like age _____ to you. [Continue with chair #2, etc.]
What's going on here?

Now begins the therapy proper. The patient might look at the situation with confusion. "It looks like a mess to me" is the most common response. "Well, are there any chairs that seem to be on one side of this conflict? If so, would you put those chairs together?" Check to make sure he has put the chairs exactly the way he wants them. "Do the position of the chairs feel exactly right to you? If not, then just change them however you wish." The client is now focusing and becoming very intent about the positioning of the chairs, thus regressing into a more concrete, childlike thinking. "What about the other chairs? Where do they belong?" Order is forming out of chaos. When this procedure is completed, then it is prudent for the therapist to understand where the problems lie and where there are resources that might help. With the transcript in the patient's hand, sitting in the appropriate chair, have him begin talking to another chair who feels quite differently from the one at hand. Stand beside the chair that is speaking to give silent support. At any time one chair speaks to another, have the patient move to the chair that is addressed. This process is now the same as dialoguing under hypnosis, mentioned in previous chapters. Each chair, using the name given by the client, needs to be heard by addressing another chair. Interaction is now occurring. Look for needs to be met within the system, and who is willing to help out whom. If a young child state cries, then it is useful to crouch down beside the chair to lower one's height, or to touch the shoulder of that feeling state. Each state needs to know that you are there, not to solve the problem, but to be a witness to it. The therapist says very little except to have the patient move from one chair to another. At some point there will be a closure, a resolution that seems satisfactory, at which time the therapist has the client stand, and asks, "How do you feel now?"

It is truly fascinating to watch people resolve their own problems with only a modicum of help from the therapist. In the many times I have given this demonstration, none were ever exactly alike, even when the problem addressed was identical. Because the process has personal meaning, it is intriguing to watch what they do with the chairs. Some stack one on top of another; others very carefully adjust the angle of one chair to the other. Another turns a chair around to denote noninvolvement in the problem. Someone else may line up several chairs behind another, explaining how they see that relationship.

The emotional reactions vary greatly. For some the whole process is intellectual. For someone else the emotions erupt like a volcanic abreaction. And sometimes the reaction is somatic. One volunteer subject at the point of anger erupted in a violent nosebleed. He didn't move, and I just stood beside him until it subsided. (Others provided towels.) It was a significant release for him.

It becomes a moot point whether or not these are truly ego states and if this is really hypnosis. With a good hypnotic subject, it appears that they enter a hypnotic state and that these feeling states seem to be well-formed ego states within their system. In a poor hypnotic subject, I believe they are just feelings that are better understood and with which the patient can come to some resolution.

In summary, here is an outline of this procedure.

PART I: Discovery of Ego State Attitudes about a Specific Problem

1. Set the stage; explain to the client that we all have mixed emotions, different parts of us feel differently, etc.

2. Decide on a topic for each ego state chair to address itself to and have it begin with "I feel . . . "

3. Have each chair express *its* position on the topic while the therapist records verbatim as much as possible. Do not suggest the sex of the ego state; let the client do it.

4. Have the client move from chair to chair until he or she cannot find another feeling state inside.

5. Sit in a chair not yet used by the patient while recording like a secretary.

PART II: Delineation of the Characteristics of Each Ego State

1. Stand beside the client, look at the appropriate chair, and read off the transcript of each feeling state with appropriate resonant voice, as the patient expressed it.

2. Have the patient give a description of each feeling state. (Don't allow negative labeling.)

3. Ask for a title or name that encapsulizes that state for the client.

4. Ask, "How old does he or she feel to you—older, younger, or contemporary?" If the client gives a noncontemporary age, then ask, "What comes to mind when you think of age (given)?"

PART III: Partnership Step

1. Place recorded notes on appropriate chairs.

2. Standing beside client, review transcript, name, age and brief description of each feeling state given by the client.

3. Ask, "How do you see what's going on here?" or words to that effect.

PART IV: Therapist Interventions

1. Follow the lead of the client. First follow, then lead in direction client seems to be going, but stay together.

2. Have client align chairs to distinguish between allies and adversaries.

3. Obtain some closure or resolution through "internal" dialoguing between states.

It is interesting to note that sometimes the client's labeling and description do not seem to fit the transcript that the client subjectively expressed while sitting in a chair. No matter. It is not the function of the therapist to point this out. The client will handle it as he or she sees fit.

This technique can be very useful unless the problem is profound and unconsciously deep-seated. After all, not every problem requires psychological unearthing. It also has the advantage of not involving the word *hypnosis*. The patient has his eyes open and is aware of his surroundings. The principles are the same as ego state therapy with hypnosis: There is the search for constructive forces, the meeting of needs within the system, the dialoguing, and the integration. The therapist is not the director of a play; in fact, the therapist allows the "play" to resolve itself with a minimum of intervention.

THEORETICAL NOTES

There are many aspects of this procedure which are like the more common ones of activating and working with ego states under hypnosis. Hypnosis is a focusing mechanism. There is increased focusing as the client moves from chair to chair.

When the patient is first sitting in a chair, and the therapist asks him to start out with "I feel . . . " she is calling for a focusing on his inner states. The things he discloses at this time may be regarded as "subject" or as experiential "self" reports. As he moves to a different chair with a different set of "I feel's," he is moving to a different aspect of his self.

During the second round the therapist has him stand up facing the chair and describe "it" from the external point of view. She is now calling for a perceptual "object" report, no longer an "*I* feel," but an "*it* appears to be."

An ego state is defined by what lies inside its boundaries versus what is outside—like a country, which is defined by its citizens (who live inside its territory) versus aliens (who live outside). From the standpoint of ego state theory (chapters 2 and 3) the verbalizations when the client is seated in a chair are "ego-cathected." When the client stands in front of a chair and describes it, his verbalized report is now "object cathected."

By a geographical focusing, as the individual sits in a chair or moves out of it, the significant ego states are delineated, similarly as they are by a hypnotic focusing. During this procedure (because it is focusing) patients sometimes actually enter light trance states, although the word "hypnosis" is not used.

This "nonhypnotic" procedure can permit a therapist who is not experienced with hypnotic procedures to practice ego state therapy. Or it can be an initial session that leads to hypnotic ego state therapy later.

11

BRIEF HYPNOANALYTIC EGO STATE THERAPY

In trying to understand how any system of therapy works, we have read many publications in which the clinicians presented case examples. These were often brief, summarized vignettes reporting the final results as judged by the therapist. However, we have frequently been disappointed that not enough tactical details and thinking of the clinician were provided for us to truly comprehend what he or she was doing—the how and why. We, too, have often followed this format in reporting earlier cases of ego state therapy (Watkins, H., 1978; Watkins, J., 1949, 1992b; Watkins & Watkins, 1979, 1981, 1982, 1986, 1991).

Accordingly, rather than present a number of cases in this work, we have opted to describe in more detail two representative ones. The first is typical of individuals who have suffered a lifelong "problem" that did not originate specifically in a severe, traumatic event, but which resulted in a chronic impairment of happiness and functioning. Often such a condition was rooted in parental neglect, misguided "discipline," and frequent humiliations from an early age. Many clients of this type, while functioning well in their careers, have frequently sought psychoanalysis and other therapies in the hope of bringing more meaning and happiness to their existences. They were not seriously ill, but they were not getting out of life what should have been possible. We shall try to present this case to give a true "flavor" of ego state therapy, including the thoughts and reactions of the therapist. This case is typical of our intensive, weekend "marathons," which we believe is a more "efficient" format, and is to be contrasted with the usual practice of once-a-week hourly sessions.

The second case, to be presented in chapter 14, is an example of a severe, lifelong one, which stemmed from violent child abuse that involved life-or-death moments, and which required many dozens of hours of ego state therapy over three years for its resolution.

Both of these cases contributed to our understanding of personality structure and theory, the psychodynamics of unconscious functioning, as well as to the development of ego state treatment techniques in our search for a more effective and efficient therapy.

If psychoanalysis and psychodynamic therapies are to be improved we might look toward their therapeutic techniques and formats, rather than to their basic theory as a hopeful possibility for change. One of these would be session frequency.

The Frequency of Sessions

In his early work Freud scheduled his patients for an hour, six days a week— and complained that "the resting day" (the Sabbath) interfered with progress of the analysis. When a day is missing, then resistance and defenses can be reinvigorated.

Today psychoanalysis usually is scheduled on a three-to-four-sessions-per-week basis, while other therapies generally schedule their patients for one session a week. If each intervening period involves the return, at least to some extent, of defenses and unresolved resistances, then treatment must be a kind of "ratcheting down" toward new and yet uncovered regions of personality. It is like moving two steps forward and one back. The next session never picks up just where the last one left off, but must first recover some of the ground already covered in the previous hour. This does not make for the greatest efficiency. On the other hand, sometimes therapy must be paced slowly for practical reasons. The optimal frequency of hours for any given type of therapy has not been determined by research, and the norms of three to five times a week in psychoanalysis, or once a week for other therapies, have crystallized more as a matter of convenience and financing. Frankly, we just don't know how often psychotherapy sessions should be held, or even whether 50 minutes is the optimum length.

The "marathon" or weekend approach, which was developed and practiced over some 20 years by Helen Watkins, seemed to get better results than the once-a-week sessions through which she treated many clients in the University of Montana's Counseling Center. Accordingly, it was adopted as the mode for most of her private practice. Moreover, the Friday-evening-to-Sunday-afternoon schedule fitted the convenience of clients from out of state, who would fly to Missoula for an intensive exposure to ego state therapy.

Most therapists schedule their patients for about an hour on a weekly basis. Such scheduling is usually convenient for both therapist and patient. And sometimes such a slow pace is necessary when gradual processing is indicated. Furthermore, this pace may fit the type of therapy being conducted, or the type of therapy with which the therapist is most familiar and comfortable. Sometimes it is desirable for the patient who might be overwhelmed by a faster pace. In other words, there are many good reasons why such a schedule might be desirable.

However, there can be a negative side to this slow pacing. Whatever progress occurred during one session may be hindered by the building up of resistance in the interim prior to the following session. Resistance, after all, is protective and a normal part of all therapy. The human organism, whether physical or psychological, is constantly trying to stabilize at homeostasis. Patterns that are familiar are less threatening than change, even if those patterns are damaging to soma or psyche. Change presents the ogre of the unknown, and what is unknown is unpredictable and therefore threatening.

In working with ego states and hypnosis, it is certainly possible to schedule appointments on a weekly basis. However, I (HHW) have gradually changed my scheduling to work at a faster pace with people who have ego state problems. I schedule them for a whole weekend, lasting approximately 10 to 15 hours. Many of my clients are therapists who were former participants in the ego state workshops that John and I conduct throughout the United States and overseas. Some clients are referred by these therapists, and occasionally the client brings along or refers a significant other.

They usually fly in Friday afternoon, whereupon I see them for two hours for history taking. The Saturday session may last four to six hours and the Sunday session usually a little less. They then return home either Sunday afternoon or Monday morning. Occasionally a Monday session is needed, but rarely. It is important that the patient feels a sense of closure. Therefore, the option of additional time is always open.

It is interesting to note how the limit of time affects the therapy. The patient is highly motivated to achieve a therapeutic goal. He or she is more likely to work hard, to take emotional risks, to trust more rapidly. The therapist is more concentrated, more tuned in, also aware that time is limited in reaching the therapeutic goal determined by the client. The experience becomes a close-working partnership.

There is also an advantage in seeing people who must travel some distance away from home. They cannot return Friday or Saturday evening to their home with differing distractions and perhaps old neurotic patterns of interaction. The weekend is just for them, no one else. It is a special time of self-exploration, conflict resolution, self-nurturance, and healing.

Occasionally, someone feels the need to resume therapy on a continuing basis with their local therapist, sometimes not. Because the weekend session is an opening-up process, it may be wise for the patient to process what has transpired with a local therapist. It is the patient, however, who is the expert on this decision. Because they have found their first experience valuable and efficient, a few clients request another weekend months or a year later in order to probe another aspect of their lives.

The most frequent comment from former patients months or even years later can be summarized as follows: "My, but that was a powerful experience!" (See chapter 13.) That expression suggests that their ego state therapy was deep and long-lasting. We have found it to be efficacious and cost effective. Insurance companies, however, are not aware of such potential economy.

A Representative Sample of Weekend Ego State Therapy

The following case involved ten therapy hours over a weekend: two hours for history-taking on Friday, five on Saturday, and three on Sunday.

My first question at the beginning of the history-taking is always, "What would you like to be able to accomplish this weekend?" This question immediately suggests that therapy is *the patient's* goal, *his or her* accomplishment, even though I am there to aid in this process. It sets the stage for partnership. It also provides a focus for both of us, a goal to reach for, and a way of evaluating what was accomplished at the weekend's end.

This patient was a 55-year-old divorced counselor (whom I shall call "Carly"), who weighed about 250 pounds and had two grown children. Carly had experienced several kinds of therapy on and off over the years, which she considered useful in differing ways. The purpose in seeing me was to be able to lose weight, to finish her Master's degree, to reduce her resistance to exercise, and to feel less alienated from people. She had tried to lose weight through many programs, each time losing but eventually adding more weight. The harder she tried, the more resistance she felt. She had nearly completed her Master's degree six years previously but lacked the equivalent of one semester's work. It would have been financially and professionally advantageous to her to have completed this degree long ago.

The purpose of the first two hours on Friday was for me to understand her background, childhood, and attitudes, and for her to become acquainted with me in order to develop mutual trust. The description of her childhood was phrased by an aunt in one word: neglect. She could not recall ever being held and hugged. She was not sexually abused, beaten, or traumatized in drastic ways, but both parents were critical and unaffectionate. Crying and anger were forbidden. After reaching high school she had to support herself. She learned to be independent and resourceful but on the inside felt lonely and alienated from the world. She was simply left to her own devices. The parents were frugal with food, especially with meat, and she felt deprived of what she wanted to eat. In junior high she recalled her mother giving her diet snacks after school, saying she was too fat, but old photographs did not reveal such a reality. Also, she heard such statements as, "Don't think you're so smart." And she was never complimented for any achievement. The only bright light on this dim horizon were both sets of grandparents who were good to her. There was little bonding with her sisters, who were three and seven years younger. After several years of marriage, when she could no longer live with a "clam" like her father, she divorced her husband.

EXERPTS FROM THERAPY SESSIONS

Saturday Session (Five Hours)

I (HHW) hypnotized Carly and led her to an oblong table in the hallucinated room (mentioned in chapter 9). I asked for anyone to come in who wished to be heard, "but if there is no one, that's just fine." The patient reported seeing a baby clinging to her.

> Therapist: She needs to know there's nothing wrong with her and that she is lovable. [Tears flow; she reports holding the baby and reassuring her.] Is there anyone else who wants to come in?
> Patient: A 6-year-old who sits across from us.
> 6-year-old: [This ego state talks to me directly.] It's not fair! Mother is mean to me; she won't let me get mad or even look mad or even cry.
> T: But you can get mad now! [6-year-old immediately expresses anger at her mother and enjoys pounding her.]

After this abreaction I have the 6-year-old notice Carly holding the baby as a good mother would.

> 6-year-old: Oh, I want her to hold me, too. [Carly does so.] It feels so nice, so different.
> T: I think Carly wants to talk to you. [In that way the hypnotized patient can say what she wishes to the 6-year-old.]
> [Long pause]
> 6-year-old: It's okay that I'm smart, she says. I don't have to pay attention to that woman who was my mother; she didn't want me. Now I have a new mother; Carly loves me.
> T: You can now be free to be you.
> 6-year-old: I think I want to get down and play.

T: Now I wonder if anyone else wants to come in, but if not that's just fine.

P: It's a teenager. She's shy. She tried to be a good girl, but it didn't do any good. She didn't know it wasn't her fault.

T: Tell us what you want, Teenager.

Teen: They're the boss. Dad gets so mad when I cry. He yells at me in his workshop. I'll get hit if I say what I want.

T: I won't let him! [I take the risk that by now I will have enough therapeutic leverage for this maneuver to be effective.]

Teen: Will you hold his arms?

T: Yes! Say whatever you want.

Teen: [To Dad] You won't listen to me. When my sister takes my clothes, you won't do anything. You're useless! I hate you; you're so mean; you're so nasty. You won't let me try things. When I do good, you won't tell me. It's always the mistakes you tell me!

T: What's wrong with being smart?

Teen: Yeah, I'm smarter than you are. You want to control everything I do. I have to learn my own things. Are you afraid I'm gonna learn that you don't know everything? [She reports father crumbling.] I think I'll sit by Carly; she knows better.

T: Hear what Carly has to say.

[Long pause for internal dialoguing]

Teen: Carly knows. She learned to know in different ways when something was right. We both know what we know. It's such a relief to be next to her.

T: Did you hold her back from finishing her Master's degree?

Teen: Yes, because the secret would be out that maybe we really *didn't* know if she wrote it down [completed graduate work]. But she's not mad at me for doing that.

T: I guess she understands you were just scared. What Carly needs from you is to believe in her.

Teen: You're right. I was in Father's camp, but now I'm in Carly's camp. Mother wouldn't help, either.

P: There's a lump in my chest [new symptom].

T: Let the lump come up in your throat.

P: Oh, it hurts so much. [Cries and moans] Something is keeping it from coming all the way out; somebody else wants to come in. Oh, there's a whole lot of them; they're all talking at once, almost chaotic, different sizes and ages. I have to extend the table; it's not long enough for everybody [concrete thinking].

T: Ask for a spokesman [to bring order out of chaos].

P: Okay, there's a young adult. The rest are not distinct. She says it's all about lost hopes. She says I know what it's all about.

T: Is the lost hope that the parents will never love you, no matter what you do? [Patient nods.] But it's not your fault because they didn't know how to love. You tried everything, but you couldn't get the love they didn't have to give. [Patient cries bitterly and deeply.]

P: My God, how strongly I hoped. I had no idea.

T: You gave up that hope with your adult self but not with your child selves.

P: [Addresses the group] Thanks for trying. You didn't know what the answer was; you just kept on trying to figure it out. [To me] It feels like they're all coming into me. [Integration?] Then I can keep trying for things I want to try, but not for that. That's why they gave up and felt like a failure; so all of them who kept on trying but couldn't make it came home now to me. Baby can feel it. She doesn't feel as helpless. She has a different energy. She's sort of looking out now; she knows it's safe to look outward. Nice. She's still in my arms and always has a place there, but she can go down if she wants. She seems bigger. She doesn't feel as needy, and I feel calmer with her.

T: Is there anyone in particular who doesn't want you to lose weight?

P: There's someone who poked her face in the door and went back.

T: Maybe she's afraid and doesn't want to be seen.

P: I think she's a baby. There seems to be another person with her. Oh, there's a whole bunch. They shake their heads with their mouths clamped shut. Lots of them are hungry. The baby was hungry for food; others for love. The baby cried for hunger and gave up 'til she didn't know any more when she was hungry. The teenager can help.

T: Maybe the teenager can feed the baby until she's satisfied.

P: There are others that want the teenager's help. They have to know that there will always be enough. They don't have to eat it up or save it in case there's not enough the next time. That's odd; there's a wall between the baby and the others. They're afraid I'll find out what they're up to and make them stop. They're afraid if they don't have enough, bad stuff will come in.

T: I'm going to shine a flashlight on the wall. Tell me what you see [mirroring her concrete thinking–projective technique].

P: Scrapes and scars; high, lava wall. All the reasons why I have to be heavy are behind the wall. Really strong. I think we'll just lean on the wall for support. See if it can learn what we know, so they don't feel threatened. I need to tell them that they'll be all right. I'm not going to tell them they're wrong, but I appreciate all they've done to help. I know they've been isolated because I've been trying to break it down, and then they made the wall thicker. Maybe there's some level of weight we need to keep, but this level is dangerous to our health. I hope they can hear me. Oh, a tiny voice just said, "We hear you." If you hear me, can we talk more? I need you. You're all part of me.

[To me] The wall is dissolving. Feels heavy in my chest. They're coming around the table. They're dark and twisted up, but they're strong—lots of energy in them.

[To those who came from behind the wall] I want to know who you are and what you are about. You are causing me more harm than what you know. It's feelings, isn't it? You make me forget when I shop. Tastiness doesn't make up for no love. You make me forget the consequences of good taste. I don't know if you know that. I know you don't mean to cause problems. You don't need to protect me like that any more. I'm strong enough to feel those feelings and be okay. I guess I want my feelings back. I want my body back.

[To me] It seems like there's four of them. [Ego states?]

T: Maybe they'll speak to you now [suggesting inner dialoguing].

P: The first one stands up. She's age 12. She's the one who came home to Rye Crisp and buttermilk after school. She doesn't know she's not fat.

T: Better tell her.

P: You're not fat. You have a little pot belly; it's just your body shape. It's in the family. It's not your fault. You didn't do anything wrong.

[To me] Seems like there's tension in her. [Cries]

12-year-old: Anything that felt good was to eat something. I knew it was wrong, so I had to hide. I couldn't help it.

T: There's nothing wrong with you.

12-year-old: Carly says there's nothing wrong with me, too. I was angry at Father but I couldn't tell him, and at Mother too. She complained about buying me big sizes. [Expresses anger at both parents and puts them down a garbage disposal.] I got rid of them so I don't have to feel not okay any more, so I don't have to eat to feel better.

T: So you and Carly can get together and find different ways to feel better.

P: There's another one, a 2-year old. I have to follow her; she's going really deep. She's remembering a time when we were little, at a gathering, dressed me up in wings like Cupid, no clothes on, felt

yucky. They all laughed. Went to bed and sucked my thumb, felt
better. I couldn't make them stop.

T: But now you can do whatever you want.

2-year-old: You took advantage of a little kid! You all laughed at me;
that made it worse. I wanted to be *big*. If I'm big, they can't do that.
Carly says she'll take care of me. She knows how not to be taken
advantage of like that.

P: There's about a 25-year-old. She feels embarrassed because as an
adult she should have known better. After my youngest was born,
everything seemed to be right in my world. I was eating healthy.
Then everything clamped down again. I caught them unawares and
they got scared. So they realized they had to watch me more closely.

T: What about the fourth one? [So far she had mentioned only three
of the four from behind the wall.]

P: It's a little child about 4 or 5, trying to look grown up, wearing a big
ferocious mask. She must be afraid. I'm going to reach out to her to
share her fear. She played doctor with a cousin. Later it felt shameful
and it became a terrible secret. She didn't tell it at confession, and it
felt like a heavy burden she had to carry around – like the weight. She
doesn't need that burden any more.

T: You don't have to carry that burden around any more.

So ended Saturday's therapy with arousal from hypnosis. Carly felt good
and encouraged as we processed the meaning of the day's session.

Saturday's Session: Summary and Analysis (JGW)

The therapist (HHW) uses a nondirective "projective" approach to activate
ego states, including the freedom to report none, if the patient wishes. The
patient (Carly) moves directly to her basic problem, a "lifelong" self-feeling of
being unlovable, and relates it to babyhood.

She next regresses to age 6 and relives (not merely remembers) indignation
at maternal rejection. She confronts her "mother representation" ego state
(an abreaction) and "enjoys pounding on her." The "baby" can now be held,
and a 6-year-old ego state wants to participate in this.

This experience is followed by a dialogue between the adult (hypnotized)
Carly and the 6-year-old in which this child state, freed through the abreact-
ion, can now accept messages of encouragement and support from the adult
Carly.

The action now moves to a teenager ego state whose feelings of inferiority relate to a critical father. The teenager (with support from the therapist) confronts the internalized father state and tells him off – thus eliminating his unconscious influence and power over Carly.

She emerges from this abreactive confrontation with enhanced self-respect. She now *knows* she is "smart," and father can no longer negate this. The teenager state moves from a past, fearful alliance with father to a supportive identification with Carly.

A painful "lump" appears, which represents repressed crying, that as a child she was not permitted to do. The therapist "invites" the lump out, and in a tearful abreaction Carly releases this pent-up emotion. She no longer needs to futilely seek her parents' love. She can love herself. The therapist provides an acceptable rationale for the parents' neglect: "because they didn't know how to love."

There is a general "integration" of the ego states into a supporting group, and Carly, now as the leader and spokesman for her entire "self," addresses them and demonstrates "love" for these previously rejected (and dissociated) parts of her self. This includes "holding the baby" ("She's still in my arms and always will have a place there").

Through a cognitive-affect bridge the therapist activates another baby state, perhaps the earlier one or maybe a different one. This baby state's problem is hunger. Apparently, as an infant Carly was insufficiently fed. This baby is walled off (dissociated) from both Carly and her other ego states. The therapist ties into the teenager ego state's rescuing need: Perhaps it will feed the baby.

The therapist, through a projective technique (flashlight) directs attention to the "wall" that dissociates the hungry baby state from the rest of Carly's self. The wall "dissolves." The baby seeks to understand and integrate with Carly and the other states ("I want my feelings back. I want my body back.")

The eating problem is reactivated by a 12-year-old state, which abreactively expresses anger at both parents and "puts them down a garbage disposal" – childlike, concrete thinking.

Next, a 2-year-old ego state remembers a humiliating experience ("wings like Cupid") where everybody made fun of Carly. It then (also abreactively) "tells off" her teasing tormentors.

Toward the end of the five-hour Saturday session a 25-year-old state begins cognitively to "integrate" newly discovered insights, concerning previously dissociated child states. The walls have dissolved.

The session finishes as Carly recalls a "shameful" experience at age 4 to 5 involving sexual experimentation.

Sunday Session (Three Hours)

Carly noticed she had not eaten all her breakfast that morning; she felt she had enough and was satisfied. She thought about the theme of holding on and letting go, not only symbolic of her weight but also of her feelings.

I hypnotized her and asked for an "Observer," if available. The finger signals indicated a "yes" but no voice. I asked it to take her wherever she needed to go to re-experience whatever was important.

P: I feel hot all over, my breathing is fast, forehead tight, dark, heart pounding, afraid, alone. [Feels around her] It's a crib! [Cries]

[I have Carly rescue her. . . . Pause]

   She feels safe now that she has a place with me. Richard, my guide, is here. He came when you called for an observer. He helps out but mostly listens.

T: Maybe he can take you wherever you need to go or whatever you need to do.

P: I need to move my body—exercise. Father said girls will develop muscles where they aren't supposed to be, so he wouldn't let me take gymnastics.

T: But you can do that now!

P: I'm going to run like the wind.

T: Go ahead: Do what you want. You'll be all right.

P: Oh, that feels so good. It's like being let out of prison!

T: The grown-up Carly knows how much exercise she can do and not hurt the body.

P: The fat helped me when I needed it, when I didn't have anything else. It kept me cozy and safe. Now I don't need it. It makes it hard to move.

T: I wonder if Richard could take you to any other place you need to go [trying to clear out any other problem that remains].

P: I'm walking down a dirt pathway with Richard, flowers on the side. The path goes down a ravine, rocky walls on each side, and a dead end with rock all around. I'm supposed to climb up; it's really steep.

T: Richard must have thought you could do it.

P: Yeah. Richard is helping me; it's a long way. Now I'm standing at the top. Looks like the Grand Canyon! Just walking along the edge a little ways. It's like saying goodbye to a place I've been for a long time. I can see all the places I tried to climb out and didn't make it. When I look away from the canyon I see all kinds of things spread out—things to look at. I want to see what's there. It looks manageable. I think I can do it. I didn't know I was in a canyon. It feels good to be up here.

T: It feels good to be free.

P: It's like standing on top of the world. There's an eagle on my left shoulder. He can fly now. He had a hard time flying in the canyon. I don't see anyone in the doorway [referring to the hallucinated room]. If there's anyone left, they can find the doorway. We'll have a place to meet. And you can be there, too.

T: Thank you. If anyone needs to contact you, you will have a meeting place?

P: Oh, I'll just know. It feels so different in my chest—no longer tight. Richard is smiling at me.

T: Who named him "Richard"?

P: He named himself. He's always been with me, but I didn't know him until I was an adult. He makes me pay attention to things when I need to. Oh, I feel in my body in one piece. I can feel all parts of my body!

Upon arousal from hypnosis Carly felt complete. We processed, reviewed, and ended our therapy. Six months later a phone call confirmed her continued feeling of togetherness and a weight loss of 20 pounds. She was also seriously planning the completion of her graduate degree as soon as finances permitted.

Sunday's Session: Summary and Analysis (JGW)

Carly shows signs of change in eating habits. An "Observer" state, "Richard," is activated (see chapter 9), who now acts as an internal "guide." He helps the child states and encourages freedom of expression (such as running). Carly symbolically walks with Richard to "the top" and surveys "the Grand Canyon" in which she had been "imprisoned" lifelong.

Carly feels "free," and can now better understand her life, since the dissociated ego states, with their fears, angers, and repressed strivings, are now consciously available. She feels integrated: "in my chest," "my body in one piece. I can feel all parts of my body." Richard remains as an internal guide and friend, available when she needs help and consultation.

Ego state therapy, using hypnoanalytic techniques, can often cross time lines rapidly, as within this five-hour session. It does not need to wait until dissociations, repressions, and many layers of normal forgetting are stripped away.

And why did we not encounter all the time-consuming resistances? Perhaps it has do to the close resonance of the clinician's therapeutic self (Watkins, J., 1976) within the regressed hypnotic relationship. Too often, the passive listening therapist may be interpreted by the patient as agreeing with uncaring, neglecting parents or their internal representations. It then takes much longer before transferences can become manifest and through interpretation be worked-through and resolved. The element of complete trust is unnecessarily postponed.

In this case the revealing analytic work was largely accomplished in the five-hour Saturday session. The three-hour Sunday term was devoted to review, working-through, and consolidation of Carly's insights.

FOLLOW-UP

A follow-up questionnaire was sent to all ego state weekend patients carried by HHW within the past 18 years. (see chapter 13) On this form, Carly (case no. 11) identified herself and reported the following:

The problem?	Lifelong, > 55 years.
Prior therapy?	9–10 years or more.
Duration-frequency?	Usually 1 a week.
Kind of therapy?	Psychoanalytic 6 years. Including cognitive and humanistic.
Results?	Lots of insight. Varying degrees of changes. Varying awareness of the deepest, most intransigent issues. Much of it somewhat helpful. Frustration at not being able to make changes I really wanted.
Number of ego state therapy hours	10.
How long since seeing Helen?	1 year.
Results of ego state therapy?	Many, and ongoing changes that occur without effort, and are "discovered" as time goes on, e.g., attitudes, sense of self, responses to stress, attack, and family issues.
Rating of treatment?	Very effective.
Changes in health, well-being, and adjustment?	Improved self-care. Positive well-being and life decisions. Better relating to others.

Comparing ego state therapy with other approaches?	It goes straight to the source/basis of the issues. Does not arouse resistances. Seems in harmony with the whole self.
As a health professional have you used ego state therapy?	Yes, with *tremendous* impact and success.

In her reported results from prior psychoanalytic and other therapies, Carly mentioned "lots of insight" and an "awareness of the deepest, most intransigent issues." However, we wonder about her meanings here of "awareness" and "insight." Apparently they did not result in her being able to make significant alterations in personality functioning and behavior at that time. Although she reported her 9–10 years of prior therapy as "somewhat helpful," she still was "frustrated" that she was not able "to make the changes [she] really wanted to make."

This case illustrates another difference between psychoanalysis and ego state therapy. As personality develops we think of new experiences being recorded "on top" of earlier ones. The 8-year-old's understandings, behaviors, and memories are later, hence "above," so that growth and development is a continuous and one-dimensional process. Accordingly, psychoanalysis has been viewed as an exploration that seeks to disclose early maladaptive, destructive factors, starting at the "top" of the developmental process, that is, the present. Through free association and interpretation of resistances the analyst and patient work their way "down" or "back" to early determining events, which then are remembered and become conscious. This permits re-interpretation, understanding, and insight. Ten-year-old experiences are remembered and accessed before 8-year-old ones, etc.

Anna Freud (1946) accused hypnosis of "by-passing the ego," with the implication that therapeutic changes are very superficial and transitory. It seems she was thinking of hypnotic suggestion. Hypnoanalysis does not "by-pass the ego." It often does bypass ego *defenses*, much like a paratrooper in modern warfare who lands behind a defended position, and makes it no longer tenable, whereas in psychoanalysis we ordinarily attack and demolish the defended position (analyze and work through the resistance) before we can proceed further. This may be very time consuming. When a defense is *hypnoanalytically* relinquished, the ego is not destroyed; it is enlarged, as it must incorporate larger "liberated" areas of personality structure.

According to ego state theory, previously nonegotized areas that are now liberated (hence, egotized) would require additional investments of ego cathexis. These are supplied by the therapist and are available because of the intense interpersonal, resonant "therapeutic self" relationship between patient and therapist (Watkins, J., 1978a). Such liberation is demonstrated in the ego state treatment of Carly.

In ego state therapy we move back and forth through age levels, seeking those that are relevant to the presenting problem. It is not like placer mining, in which much material that is not "pay dirt" must be excavated. It is more like shaft mining. It will be noted that in Carly's Saturday session this back-and-forth movement proceeded as follows:

The center of analytic attention (after a nonpressure invitation by the therapist) moved to an infant state. Next a 6-year-old state was activated, followed by a teenager, then a fractional state described as a "lump," then back to the present-day Carly.

A new baby state appeared, which was "hungry." The problem of mother not feeding the child was then addressed through an abreacting telling-off of mother. Then back to teenager to get more help for baby, followed by the 12-year-old renewal of the hunger problem. After an "insightful" understanding by a 25-year-old state, the therapy returned to the adult, present-day Carly.

The Sunday session was devoted primarily to review and "intelligence-gathering." The observer state, Richard, could inform as to other areas that needed working-through, and since it is ageless, could help other ego states at all age levels. It was left as a permanent internal support system.

In hypnoanalytic ego state therapy we are constantly moving back and forth between activating regressed states, lifting repressed material, analyzing meanings, then contacting and integrating with the normal, egotized executive state of the patient.

Carly's case is interesting, not only as an example of ego state therapy, but because it also offers many perspectives about personality functioning, theory, and therapeutic technique.[1]

12

OUTCOME RESEARCH IN PSYCHOTHERAPY

During the last century many approaches to psychological treatment have been advocated. In these pages we have tried to present a system of psychotherapy that involves a number of techniques drawn from many sources but integrated within a theoretical framework.

Thirty-five years ago, one of us (Watkins, J., 1960) tried to collate all the systems and approaches that had been published in book form. It was a kind of personal search for "the perfect therapy." Other approaches, whose only exposure had been in article form, were probably overlooked. This project, undertaken over some eleven years, involved the reading and annotating of approximately a thousand books, followed by an outlining of each system (Watkins, J., 1993b). Ten years later, with a colleague, we tried to bring that work up to date. After an extensive library and computer research, we found it would require the reading of at least 3,000 texts to cover the field. We abandoned the project. Now in 1997 there has been added a still further mountain of thinking, research, reports, and proposals in the general field of psychotherapy.

Most of the approaches that have been proposed were developed by individual therapists who described their cases, illustrated their techniques, and sometimes presented a unique theoretical rationale for their procedures. Many simply proposed a variation of some larger and well-known system of therapy, such as behavioral, cognitive (Wright, Thase, Beck, & Ludgate, 1993), humanistic-existential, or psychoanalytic. Rarely was any objective follow-up of cases undertaken. In general, each technique or system was presented as an improvement on other approaches to psychotherapy, many self-claimed to be the best of therapies.

Ego state therapy runs the risk of being simply another such attempt, whose new contribution is questionable, and which in time after a decline in early enthusiasm will take its place on the storage shelf of therapies that have had their day, been fully explored, and at least partially discarded. As science moves forward in this area, almost certainly it will be superseded by improvements in ways of treating the psychologically impaired.

Recently, there has been a resurgence of interest by psychologists in efforts to validate psychotherapy (see American Psychological Association, 1996). Researchers today have been trying to specify a list of empirically validated therapies (Goldfried & Wolfe, 1996). Such endeavors are heartily supported by the insurance industry. Managed care and other providers want to know before funding any approach whether it is effective, for what conditions, and practiced by whom? They would like specific information on what kind or system of therapy is best for what conditions—as are known in the area of physical medicine.[1]

Securing such information scientifically is not an easy task in the realm of psychological treatment. First, it is difficult to know just what constitutes improvement in mental health, and how it can be measured. Must we rely exclusively on the subjective reports of patients, "I feel better?" Or can we find objective criteria, perhaps couched in specific terms, such as, "I am now able to go to work, whereas before treatment I was unable to function on the job?" Current studies have approached the problem generally from one of two basic designs: efficacy and effectiveness.

Efficacy (sometimes called clinical trials) refers to the results of a systematic evaluation of the intervention in a controlled clinical research. This type of study tests the effect of specific procedures under laboratory conditions, such as a specified number of sessions, on volunteers who are presumed to represent a randomized sample of the population to which the treatment procedure will be applied (Barlow, 1996). Findings from efficacy studies are said to be empirically based. Therapists tend to criticize such studies as mechanical, manual-based, and not applicable in the clinical situation where the therapist usually employs a wide variety of techniques and the treatment is of indeterminate length.

Effectiveness studies (called clinical utility studies by some researchers, e.g., Jacobson & Christensen, 1996) are observational (or correlational) investigations of therapy in the naturalistic treatment setting on real patients and with flexibility in procedures—as commonly occurs in clinical practice. Evaluation studies are usually follow-up measures involving self-reports by patients concerning their reactions to their treatment, although some aim at external observations of subsequent patient behaviors. Experimentalists claim that such studies are not truly empirical and cannot measure cause and effect. Furthermore, self-reports can be criticized as being subject to many biases, such as malingering, desire to please the doctor, etc. Both approaches have limitations and suffer from design flaws.

There have been numerous studies on outcome research in general and many comparing the effectiveness of various approaches (Bergin & Lambert, 1978; Claghorn, 1976; Frank, 1979; Landman & Dawes, 1982; Seligman, 1995; Smith & Glass, 1981). *Consumer Reports* has recently undertaken a very comprehensive, follow-up study on the effectiveness of their treatment as reported by subscribers who had experienced psychotherapy.

The *Consumer Reports* study (1995), which involved questionnaire replies from 7,000 subscribers, had the advantage of studying psychotherapy as it is actually practiced in the field, hence, in the real-life situation. The general findings were as follows:

- Psychotherapy was a positive benefit to patients.
- Long-term therapy did better than short-term treatment.
- All of the major systems (cognitive, behavioral, humanistic, and psychoanalytic) had about equal results.[2]
- Patients whose time of care or choice of therapist was limited by insurance or managed care didn't do as well.

This research was evaluated by Seligman (1995) in terms of its methodological virtues and drawbacks as contrasted with more traditional efficacy studies. He concluded that the design, although it could be improved, was essentially sound and relevant, and that its "underlying survey method provides a powerful addition to what we know about the effectiveness of psychotherapy." It presented compelling proof that, in general, psychotherapy works. People are helped by such treatment.

Not all researchers agreed with Seligman's conclusions. The *Consumer Reports* study stimulated heated controversy on the problems in evaluating the effectiveness of psychotherapy (see Barlow, 1996; Goldfried & Wolfe, 1996; Hollon, 1996; Howard, Moras, Brill, Martinovich, & Lutz, 1996; Jacobson & Christensen, 1996; Newman & Tejeda, 1996; Sechrest, McKnight, & McKnight, 1996; Seligman, 1996; Strupp, 1996).

The practice of psychotherapy today, more than previously, is facing a serious challenge. Psychological treatment, like medical treatment, is currently being financed primarily by insurance companies and other third-party payers. These organizations are not willing to fund treatments that require several sessions a week over many months, and often years. They insist on brief, effective, "efficient" methods. The risk is that quality and long-lasting effects of treatment will be sacrificed for low-cost, temporary symptom alleviation.

Many of these and other studies have tried to measure the efficacy of some specific therapeutic approach or technique, behavior therapy and cognitive therapy being the most commonly studied. Behavior therapy has appealed to both researchers and insurance payers because it is specific, can be evaluated objectively, and seems to be a technique which is relatively independent of the skill and experience of the therapist. Behavior therapy has long been proven effective by many studies for such issues as weight control and stop smoking, and specific conditions such as phobias (see Turner, Calhoun, & Adams, 1981).

Cognitive therapy (Beck, 1983) has been shown effective in the treatment of neurotic depressions and, like psychoanalysis, it does so through an achieving of "insight." However, like bits of a jigsaw puzzle already laid out, the cognitive therapy approach seeks to find a meaningful pattern to those pieces of which the patient is already consciously aware. It does not probe for deeper and "unconscious" matters of which the patient had previously been unaware—as do psychoanalytic, hypnoanalytic, and other psychodynamic approaches. It is usually much briefer than psychoanalysis, but its effectiveness with lifelong disturbances, rooted in repressed and traumatic childhood events, has not yet been determined.

We hope that psychotherapy research will be continued, and that our seminal work here in ego state therapy will stimulate investigators to include this approach among their research targets. However, we also agree with Strupp (1996) when he points out that "the critical feature of all successful therapy, it seems to me, is the therapist's skillful management of the patient-therapist relationship," and that this encompasses "such qualities as the ability to listen empathically, a caring attitude, warmth, compassion and commitment to patients' welfare. Unfortunately, very few of the studies reported have paid any attention to the "person or self" of the therapist as a therapeutic agent, probably because these factors cannot be conveniently measured by experimental controls. We may study therapy as a *science*, but we practice it as an *art*.

Psychoanalytically oriented practitioners believe that permanent progress in patients requires significant personality reorganization. This involves insight into causative factors. A psychodynamic therapy, incorporating the aims of psychoanalysis, but able to achieve these in a much shorter time, is badly needed, but it must be able to demonstrate long-term effectiveness as well as short-term efficiency.

Any technique, approach, or system of treatment is applied by a therapist who is a human being. And people vary widely from each other. There is no skill practiced by humans in which the effectiveness of the various prac- titioners do not widely differ: baseball, painting, speaking, writing, etc. A therapy technique is like an instrument used in the hands of a person. Deter- mining its effectiveness is like asking whether a violin makes good music when played. An improved therapy technique, like an improved violin, such as a Stradivarius, should indeed get better results. However, in the hands of Isaac Stern it is not the same instrument as in those of a young, beginning fiddler— even though the novice holds the instrument according to the printed direc- tions in a manual or instruction book. We believe this to be true of every approach to psychotherapy. Theodore Reik practiced with a "third ear" (1948) in a much different way from the average new graduate of a psychoana- lytic institute.

Throughout all our experience and previous writings we have insisted that the person of the therapist, not the technique, is *the most significant variable* in determining success or efficiency of an approach.[3] Accordingly, every person being different, we are confronted with an almost impossible task of trying to measure the relative effectiveness of an approach as compared to others. Are results achieved in a case due to the type of therapy, its theoretical founda- tions, its techniques, or the competence of its practitioner? Even the most objective of procedures, such as the giving of a pill or the applying of a positive reinforcement in a behavior-therapy sequence, can vary depending on who gives it. Furthermore, therapists do not always practice exactly as they say they do.

Some years ago, while teaching a graduate course in general psychotherapy, I (JGW) collected a number of audiotapes from well-known and widely pub- lished psychotherapists, psychoanalysts, cognitive therapists, behaviorists, hu- manistic practitioners, etc. I had my students listen to them as presumed exemplifications of reality therapy, psychoanalysis, Jungian analytic therapy, Gestalt therapy, Adlerian individual therapy, client-centered (nondirective) therapy, and many others. They were asked to read books and articles on these approaches, study outlines of the various procedures (Watkins, J., 1960), and listen to the tapes, many from very prestigious practitioners who made recordings of their treatment sessions.

Students complained bitterly. All too often they felt that the practitioner simply did not follow the principles and techniques he or she had advocated and published. When it came to actual recordings of what transpired during the therapeutic sessions, theory and practice departed widely. There was also a leveling in that many who claimed to have an approach that was quite unique did not in their actual handling with patients seem to be very much different from other clinicians who presented themselves as practicing a differ- ent system.

Assessments of therapeutic effectiveness are further clouded, not only by who did the treatment and utilized the stated approach, but also by who did the follow-up evaluation. Therapists have stakes in the procedures they advocate and publish. It is human for them to want their patients to report improvement – perhaps "cure." This serves as a built-in bias, which leaves their reports of the success of their own treatment suspect. Our attempt here to follow-up our ego state patients may certainly be subject to the same criticism.

To truly assess the effectiveness of ego state therapy would require that we do extensive pre- and postevaluations of many therapists (who presume to practice as ego state therapists) of the amount of time involved, the severity of the conditions being treated, and many other factors. This would require, perhaps, a large grant-supported study, several years of time, and significant university resources.

Unfortunately, we both are retired from academia and cannot now undertake such a project. However, we do have some data from which tentative findings might be derived, and it is from such a perspective that we have sought some objective evaluation of the effectiveness and efficiency of ego state therapy.

Is it a new approach, or simply a rehash, a different combination of that which has already been proposed, explored, and tested? Perhaps more cogent is not whether it is something new, but is it effective as a treatment for the kinds of conditions for which it is recommended? If effective, is it an improvement on, or more efficient than, other well-known and widely practiced approaches, psychoanalytic therapy, behavioral, cognitive, or humanistic therapy? Does it have anything unique to add to the present wealth of human experience in the treatment of psychological ills?

Seligman's (1995) evaluation of the *Consumer Reports* study has many valuable suggestions for future research in the effectiveness of therapy, involving better controls and improved experimental design. While we cannot do the all-encompassing and compelling study on effects we would like to do, we can at least report an attempt on our part to gather some relatively objective data about the patients treated over the past 15–20 years. We make no claim that the patients reported in this study are representative, or even that our ego state therapy was the only significant factor in their subsequent improvement or change of condition. The study constituted an objective questionnaire sent to all the patients who within the past 18 years had received intensive therapy from one of us, HHW, primarily according to her model of the "marathon" weekend as described and illustrated in chapter 11.

These patients were not representative of those who seek psychological treatment because of severe and incapacitating psychopathologies. They were largely mental health professionals, psychologists, psychiatrists, plus family members and patients of the foregoing. They felt the need for personal therapy because of "problems." But most of them had also had extended periods of personal therapy, prior to their ego state therapy sessions, such as psychoanalysis and other approaches. They did have some basis for comparison. The following describes the way in which the survey was conducted.

A questionnaire and accompanying instruction sheet was mailed to each client who had been treated by Helen during the past 18 years (in the weekend, "marathon" format) and asked to answer it anonymously. No attempt was made at that time to check on which client returned which questionnaire. It was more important that each individual feel complete privacy and confidentiality, and also be free to submit negative or critical appraisals. We did not want it to be simply an expedition to secure flattery or pleasurable satisfaction on our part. Such responses might well represent merely a wish by clients not to offend the therapist with whom they may still have positive feelings. We hoped for as complete objectivity as possible.

Accordingly, the findings reported in chapter 13 represent the patient-reported results of one therapist using ego state therapy during intensive individual weekend sessions. These results, therefore, may be ascribed to the weekend marathon scheduling, the hypnotic modality, the perspective of ego state theory, the use of ego state therapy techniques, the selectivity of the patients, the skill and sensitivity of the therapist—or any combination of these. They do not constitute a clear-cut test of the validity of ego state therapy alone. They do suggest what is possible.

13

The Effectiveness and Efficiency of Ego State Therapy: A Study in Validation

Weekend ego state therapy is a more intensive experience than once-a-week traditional treatment. It is like a "psychological surgery" aimed at resolving or extirpating a specific conflict or pathology as compared to a "spaced medication" approach in a physical disorder. The intensive marathon-weekend approach, on which the data is presented in this chapter,[1] involves accessing and integrating within a short time a great deal of (repressed) material.

Most of these patients fly in from out of state for the weekend of therapy. Accordingly, when first scheduled, they are advised to have a "resident therapist" to whom they can go subsequently for support, working-through, or follow-up if needed. Often they are referred to Helen by long-term personal therapists to whom they returned.

In order to study more objectively the results of this ego state therapy, I (JGW) decided to send out a questionnaire to Helen's previous patients. The basic purpose of the questionnaire was to try to make some objective determination of the validity of the ego state approach, its effectiveness and efficiency, especially as compared to other therapies experienced by these clients.

Since the ego state therapy cases that had been treated by JGW often involved true multiple personalities, and were not scheduled as intensive weekend marathons, they were not included in this study. Data was secured from and evaluated on only those that met the following criteria:

162

- They were seen by Helen (HHW).
- They were seen only in intensive weekend marathon sessions (8–15 hours).
- Ego state therapy was an essential part of their treatment.

A total of 86 cases, seen from 1976 through 1995, met the above criteria, and accordingly were sent the questionnaire. The questionnaire requested feedback from all who had been treated by either of us in order to minimize the personality factor, but they were sent only to patients of Helen's. Forty-six (53%) completed questionnaires were returned.

QUESTIONNAIRE ON EGO STATE THERAPY

1. What was the reason for which you entered therapy? _____
   _____
2. How long had there been a problem? _____
3. Before seeing either John or Helen Watkins in Ego State Therapy did you have any prior psychotherapy? _____
4. If "yes," what kind? Psychoanalytic _____ Cognitive _____
   Behavioral _____ Humanistic _____
   Other _____
5. Approximately how many sessions (hours)? _____
   Over how long a period? Months _____ years _____
6. Results: _____
7. How do you rate *that* treatment? Very Effective _____
   Somewhat _____ Slightly _____ Ineffective _____
8. Did it meet your expectations? Yes _____ Largely _____
   Partially _____ Very little _____ No _____
9. Add anything here you wish to describe it _____
   _____
10. How many sessions (or hours) did you have of ego state therapy with Helen Watkins _____ or John Watkins _____?
11. Were these concentrated in weekends? Yes _____ No _____
    How many weekends? _____
12. How long has it been since you saw either Helen or John Watkins in therapy? _____

13. What was the basic reason for consulting Helen or John?

_____

14. Results: _____

15. How do you rate *this* treatment? Very effective _____
    Somewhat _____ Slightly _____ Ineffective _____

16. Did it meet your expectations: Yes _____ Largely _____
    Partially _____ Very little _____ No _____

17. Add anything here you wish to describe it. _____

_____

18. Since undergoing ego state therapy has your health, well-being, and/or adjustment changed in any way? Please describe. _____

_____

19. Can you compare ego state therapy with any other approach, either which you have experienced or have knowledge of? _____

_____

20. Have you had psychotherapy with others since your sessions with Helen or John Watkins? _____ Describe. _____

_____

21. If you are a health professional, have you used ego state therapy since your work with Helen or John? _____

A FOLLOW-UP QUESTIONNAIRE ON THE EFFECTS OF EGO STATE THERAPY[2]

We have been asked to describe the ego state approach to treatment in many scientific journals and at numerous professional meetings here and abroad. While we feel that it has been helpful to most clients, we do not have the objective, scientific data on its results that are requested by professionals. That is why we are sending out this questionnaire.

The data from this inquiry are for research purposes only. Accordingly, no person will be identified, by name, by initials, or by any identifying circumstances of time, geography, etc. Every person's identity will be kept completely confidential. Your complete candor will be greatly appreciated.

The findings will be published in the form of totals and some descriptions of the treatment of those of you who give us permission to do so, but always with your privacy paramount.

We are contacting every individual who has come to us for such treatment within the past 18 years, and who did receive ego state therapy. As one of those people we will greatly appreciate your participation in this study so that we can improve ego state therapy and its theory, and in the hope that your experience will make it possible for us and others in the healing professions to offer more effective and rapid treatment.

With kind regards,

Helen H. Watkins (signed)

John G. Watkins (signed)

As questionnaires were returned, it became obvious that certain items could have been more clearly worded. For example, item 21 asked if the respondent had been a mental health professional and had then used ego state therapy after his or her personal therapy sessions. The question is somewhat ambiguous. Although many answered "yes," I did not know whether a "no" response indicated they were not a health professional, or a professional who did not use ego state therapy subsequent to their therapy with Helen. Several reported they were already familiar with this approach and had been using it previously with their own clients.

The "Problem" or Reason for Entering Therapy

In most cases the "problem" that impelled them to seek therapy (their response to item 1 or item 13) was the same. A few said they had in general resolved their initial problems, but felt that something was missing, something was still unresolved.

Some of the problems were stated in a few short terms, like "depression"; others gave rather lengthy descriptions, which we have shortened to capture their essence in briefer form. A few presented a psychiatric diagnosis. Item 2 (duration) is recorded with exact quotes. Table 1 presents the problems for which they first entered therapy and their duration as reported on the questionnaires. Table 2 summarizes the reasons for which therapy was sought.

Some respondents listed more than one problem. It is evident that in general the conditions treated were not simple transitory disturbances, but chronic ones from which many clients had suffered over a long period of time. A breakdown (difficult to tabulate because of different terms in reporting) is presented in table 3.

Prior Psychotherapy

The respondents' prior experience in personal therapy was of interest (42 had experience, 4 did not), including type, duration, and results. They obviously felt the need for further work. Many of them had taken ego state workshops with us and had seen and heard taped excerpts from our earlier cases. Moreover, those who had had such a workshop experience previously (the majority

TABLE 1

Item No. 1. The Problem: Reason Client Entered Therapy
Item No. 2. Duration of the Problem

CASE NO.[3]

1. Frequent experiences of sinking self-esteem.
   "Forever"

2. Resolve childhood traumas affecting current relationships.
   "45 years"

3. Performance anxiety. Math block. Later diagnosed dyslexia.
   "High school on" "1984"

4. Infertility, marital discord, depression.
   "2-1/2 years"

5. General understanding of integration. Migraines.
   "1983"

6. Sexual abuse memories. Lifelong depression.
   "30 years"

7. Mid-life depression. Relationship failures. Low self-esteem.
   "Lifelong"

8. Depression.
   "Several years"

9. Anxiety
   "All my life"

10. Begin to treat MPDs. Explore dissociation.
    "No known problem"

11. To resolve longstanding inner conflicts.
    "Lifelong- >55 years"

12. Depression.
    No duration listed

13. Marital problem.
    "2–5 years"

14. Irrational overreaction, anger. Anxiety, insecurity.
    "Lifelong"

15. To understand better the source of my emotions.
    "Not truly a problem"

16. Polyfragmented MPD.
    "Lifelong"

(Table 1, continued)

17. Informed about ego state therapy at your workshop.
    "From youth" (interest in exploring self)

18. Resolution of childhood trauma. Explore relationships.
    "1 year that I was firsthand aware of"

19. Understanding of personal dynamics–and wanted more.
    "Always" (sought self-understanding)

20. Unable to form a lasting love relationship.
    "Life?"

21. Stop eating compulsively and lose weight.
    "Since age 12"

22. Childhood amnesia.
    "Forever"

23. (No answer)

24. Excessive drinking.
    "10 years"

25. Blank spaces in my memories. Severe depression.
    "Years"

26. Lack of self-acceptance. Body-esteem problem.
    "20 years"

27. General performance anxiety. Neurotic depression.
    "College and twenties"

28. Abuse as a child.
    "Aware of problem a year or so before calling Helen"

29. Guilt. History of drug abuse. Sexual acting out.
    "Since age 22"

30. Child molestation. Fear of being alone. Excessive anxiety.
    "25 years +"

31. To fight cancer. Finding cause. Ensure not creating more.
    "Diagnosed Aug. 1991"

32. Healing from aftereffects of child abuse.
    "35–40 years"

33. Depression and anxiety.
    "6 months"

34. Anorgasmia and insomnia.
    "Lifelong"

continued

(Table 1, continued)

35. Unsolved dissociative symptoms related to childhood traumas.
       "Age 9"

36. Deep, powerful depression—mildly suicidal, black funk.
       "Since infancy"

37. Early attitudes re. mother. A hurt ego state was affecting relationships.
       "Adolescence–adulthood"

38. Greater relaxation and freedom to be me.
       "50 years"

39. Depression.
       "6 months"

40. Lingering doubts about possible childhood abuse.
       "20 years"

41. Obesity. Eating addiction. Afraid of intimacy.
       "Lifelong"

42. Relationship with my lover and myself in life.
       "3 to 4 months"

43. Depression and anxiety.
       "Since adolescence"

44. Preparation for marriage and parenting.
       "Since divorce" (two years ago)

45. Possible raise to consciousness of child abuse memories.
       "Have dim, vague memories confirmed or resolved"

46. Depression and aggression/sexual problem.
       "4 years"

---

of them but not all) were also familiar with ego state theory, which conceptualized this approach. They knew something of what to expect. But this would also be true of mental health professionals who undertook any other personal therapy.

Table 4 lists the types of prior therapy, frequency, and duration as reported by respondents; table 5 gives an overall summary.

It is evident from table 4 that most of the clients (42 out of 46) had previously experienced some type of psychotherapy, and that for the majority (27) it was psychoanalysis or psychodynamic in nature. Many had also experienced other kinds of therapy, such as humanistic (20) or cognitive (12). The respondents, therefore, having had much experience with many types of

TABLE 2

Summary of Reasons for which Therapy was Sought
(Items 1 and 13)

Depression	12	Emotional problems	3
Childhood	10	*anger*	
traumas		Dissociation	2
abuse		Performance anxiety	2
amnesia			
Self-	6	Compulsions	2
esteem		*eating, weight reduction*	
understanding		Addictions	2
Anxiety	5	*alcohol, drugs*	
insecurity		"Inner conflicts"	1
Marital	4	Relations with parents	1
love relationships		"Migraines"	1
Sexual problems	4	Cancer	1
impotence, frigidity			
infertility			
acting out			

TABLE 3

Summary of Problem Durations

LONG-LASTING:		
"Lifelong," "Forever," "Since infancy," "All my life," "20 years or greater," etc.	23	(50%)
INTERMEDIATE (2–19 YEARS, OR INDEFINITE):		
"1983," "2-1/2 years," "Years," "Several years," "2–5 years," "10 years," "College and twenties," etc.	15	(33%)
RECENT (LESS THAN 2 YEARS):		
"1991," "1 year," "6 months"	3	(7%)
MISCELLANEOUS:		
"No problem," "Not truly a problem" (sought for training?), or unanswered.*	5	(10%)
Total	46	

*Helen reported that a few said they came simply for ego state experience. However, in actual therapy almost all of them found and studied real, personal problems.

169

TABLE 4

Types of Prior Therapy and Frequency, Duration (Items 4, 5)

CASE NO.
1. Psychoanalytic (20 years)
2. Psychoanalytic (10 years). Humanistic, hypnotherapy
3. Humanistic, hypnosis (off and on)
4. Cognitive (2-1/2 years, once weekly)
5. Humanistic (20 sessions, 2 years)
6. Humanistic (8 years)
7. Cognitive, behavioral, hypnotherapy (3 years, 20 years ago)
8. Psychoanalytic, humanistic (100 hours, 2 years)
9. Cognitive (75 hours, 1 year, 6 months)
10. Psychodynamic (30 sessions, 8 months)
11. Psychoanalytic (6 years), cognitive, humanistic (9–10 years)
12. Psychoanalytic, humanistic (150 hours, 2-1/2 years)
13. No prior psychotherapy
14. Sulivanian, cognitive, systemic (250 hours, 2–3 years)
15. No prior psychotherapy
16. Psychoanalytic, cognitive, humanistic (0–4/week, 9 years)
17. Psychoanalytic, family therapy (7 years)
18. Humanistic (6–8 hours, 2 months)
19. Psychoanalytic (approximately 20 years)
20. Psychoanalytic, humanistic (25 years on and off since 1947)
21. Psychoanalytic (50 hours), humanistic (40 hours), group (30)
22. Eclectic transpersonal (1 hour/week, 2-1/2 years)
23. No prior psychotherapy
24. Humanistic (30 hours, 1 year)
25. Psychoanalytic (once a week, 16–18 years)
26. Psychoanalytic-humanistic (150 hours?, on and off past 8 years)
27. Psychoanalytic (2 years), humanistic, cognitive, (age 30 to 45)
28. Psychoanalytic (3 times a week, 4-1/2 years)
29. Psychoanalytic (150 hours, 3–4 years)
30. Psychoanalytic, cognitive, humanistic, (500 hours, 10 years)
31. Humanistic (30 hours, 2 years)
32. Humanistic, hypnotherapy, groups (5 + years)
33. Humanistic (80 hours, 6 years)
34. Bioenergetics (2 per week, total unknown–10 years at least)
35. Psychoanalysis (2 years), psychodynamic (9 years)
36. Psychoanalytic, behavioral, child (over 500 hours, 38 years)

(Table 4, continued)

37. Humanistic, psychodynamic, object relations (3 years)
38. Psychoanalytic, humanistic, self psychology (6–8 years)
39. Psychoanalytic (once a week, 2 years), humanistic (10 years)
40. Psychoanalytic, cognitive, behavioral (200 hours, 5 years)
41. No prior psychotherapy
42. Psychoanalytic, cognitive (12 hours, 2 months)
43. Psychoanalytic (5 years)
44. Psychoanalytic, cognitive, Jungian hypnosis (15 hours, 18 months)
45. Psychoanalytic, (440 hours, 3-1/2 years)
46. Cognitive, hypnotherapy (10 hours, 4 months)

therapies, from both firsthand experience and professional training (most of them practicing therapists themselves), were in a good position to evaluate the effectiveness of the ego state treatment they had undergone with Helen, and to compare it with psychoanalytic and other approaches.

Item 6 called for a qualitative response on results of prior therapy. Responses often contained comments like, "Modest help," "Helpful, but a feeling of something yet to be done," "Increased awareness," "Did not get to major issue," "Unfinished business," "Better cognitive understanding but not enough heart/mind change." In some cases the previous therapy was reported as "excellent" and "life-saving." In a few cases the responses were negative.

TABLE 5

Summary of Types of Prior Therapy*

Psychoanalytic (psychodynamic, object relations)	27	Bio-energetics	1
		Child therapy	1
Humanistic	20	Eclectic-transpersonal	1
Cognitive	12	Family therapy	1
Hypnotherapy	4	Jungian hypnosis	1
Behavioral	3	Sullivanian	1
Group	2	Systemic therapy	1
Total reporting prior therapy			42
Median number of sessions (hours), range 19–500+			145
Median time, range 2 months to 38 years			2 years

*Some respondents listed more than one prior therapy.

Criticisms centered around intellectuality of insight (cognitive) and length of time to get results. If the respondents' prior therapy had been completely successful they probably would not have undertaken more (ego state) therapy.

Comparison of Prior Therapy with Ego State Therapy

Item 7 asked the respondents to rate the effectiveness of their prior therapies, and item 15 asked for a rating on their ego state therapy with HHW. In table 6 the results of both are presented to permit a comparison.

A chi-square test of the difference between effectiveness of prior therapies and ego state therapy showed a significant superiority (χ^2 (2) = 15.48, p < .005) for ego state therapy.[4]

Item 8 asked respondents to rate the extent to which their prior therapies met expectations, and item 16 asked for the same judgment on their ego state therapy. In table 7 the results of both are presented for comparison.

A chi-square test of the difference between ego state therapy and prior therapies in terms of the extent to which each met client expectations showed a significant superiority (χ^2 (2) = 21.56, p < .005) for ego state therapy.[5]

The reports of those who answered the follow-up questionnaire indicated that they regarded ego state therapy more effective than their prior therapies, as summarized in table 6, and that ego state therapy met their expectations better than their former therapies, as summarized in table 7. These data, however, involved so many different therapeutic approaches that they gave us no way of directly comparing ego state therapy with any one specific system.

TABLE 6

The Rated Effectiveness of Prior Therapies (Item 7) and
Ego State Therapy (Item 15)

	PRIOR THERAPIES	EGO STATE THERAPY
Very effective	11	29
Somewhat effective	22	9
Slightly effective	4	4
Ineffective	5	0
Total	42	42

TABLE 7

The Extent to which Prior Therapies (Item 8) and Ego State
Therapy (Item 16) Met Client Expectations

	PRIOR THERAPIES	EGO STATE THERAPY
"Beyond" (written in)		1
"Exceeded" (written in)		1
Yes	7	22
Largely	8	11
Partially	18	4
Very little	5	1
No	3	2
Total	42	42

Ratings by Respondents whose Prior Therapy was Psychoanalytic

Twenty-seven of the 46 respondents reported that their prior treatment approach had been primarily psychoanalytic. The total number of sessions and/or the session frequency per week ranged from 12 to 500+, with a median of 150, over a period of from 2 months to 38 years, with a median of 5 years. Five also reported frequencies ranging from 1 per week to 4 per week, with a median of 3 per week.

These data offered a reasonable opportunity to compare their experiences in psychoanalytic therapy with those in ego state therapy. Note that due to the wording of the questionnaire, respondents could not distinguish between traditional psychoanalysis, which is usually conducted with a frequency of several sessions a week, and psychoanalytic therapy, which typically involves a single session a week and with lesser goals. However, both of these (and also ego state therapy) aim at similar objectives, namely, the reduction of neurotic, psychosomatic, and behavioral maladjustments indirectly by lifting repressions, resolving defenses, achieving insight into unconscious motivations, and developing greater, long-lasting maturity in character structure.

The differences between ego state therapy and the psychoanalytic therapies, therefore, lay primarily in the modifications of ego state *theory* (Federn's and ours) to psychoanalytic conceptions, the addition of numerous, additional techniques (made available through hypnoanalysis) and, in the cases here described, the intensive weekend "marathon" format.

TABLE 8

The Effectiveness of Prior Psychoanalytic Therapy (Item 7) and Subsequent Ego State Therapy (Item 15), as Rated by Clients Who had Experienced Both

	PSYCHOANALYTIC THERAPY	EGO STATE THERAPY
Very effective	7	21
Somewhat effective	16	5
Slightly effective	2	1
Ineffective	2	0
Total	27	27

Accordingly, the data from the 27 cases who had reported that their prior therapy was primarily psychoanalytic, were reanalyzed (see tables 8 and 9).

A chi-square test of the difference between effectiveness of psychoanalytic therapy and ego state therapy showed a significant superiority (χ^2 (3) = 14.56, p < .005) for ego state therapy.[6]

A chi square test of the difference in the extent to which psychoanalytic therapy and ego state therapy met expectations by clients who had experi-

TABLE 9

The Extent to which Prior Psychoanalytic Therapy (Item 8) and Subsequent Ego State Therapy (Item 15) Met Expectations, as Rated by Clients Who Had Experienced Both

	PSYCHOANALYTIC THERAPY	EGO STATE THERAPY
"Beyond" (written in)		1
"Exceeded" (written in)		1
Yes	4	14
Largely	8	6
Partially	13	5
Very little	1	0
No	1	0
Total	27	27

enced both showed a significant superiority for ego state therapy[7] (χ^2 (3) = 15.48, p < .005).

Frequency and Recency of Ego State Therapy

Clients who took more than a single marathon weekend did so about one year apart. Table 10 shows the number of weekend sessions as well as the recency to last contact with Helen.[8]

TABLE 10

Frequency of Ego State Therapy (Item 11) and
Time since Most Recent Weekend Ego State
Therapy* (Item 12)

Frequency			
1 Weekend	41		
2 Weekends	2		
3 Weekends	2		
4 Weekends	1		

| | *Recency* | | |
YEARS	NO.	MONTHS	NO.
"Years"	1	10	1
"Several" (years)	1	8	1
"A few years"	1	7	4
17	1	6	2
10	1	5	1
"8 or more"	1	3	1
6–8	1	2	3
6	1	1	1
5	1	Total:	46
3+	2	Median = 2 years	
3	5		
2–3	1		
2+	1		
"2 or more"	2		
2	4		
1	8		

*In cases that had more than one weekend of therapy, the time reported was for the most recent session.

Clients' Reasons for Seeking Ego State Therapy

In replying to item 13 many respondents simply reiterated their response to item 1 (why they initially entered therapy). Some, especially those not fully satisfied with their prior treatment, made comments related to trying something new or different. Several referred to a workshop they had taken with us. Some said they had been referred by a personal therapist or another mental health practitioner. A few mentioned being impressed by the personality of the therapist, HHW (as observed when taking a workshop with us). One simply said "trust." And several replied they were curious about ego state therapy, and that for both personal and professional reasons they wanted to experience it.

Construction of a Rating (Grading) System

To measure the effectiveness of the treatment received by these clients (combining *all* objective and subjective data available on the questionnaires), to compare their relative results, and then to compare with other therapies, some kind of objective rating needed to be devised. Since different clients reported the results of their therapy in different words, a qualitative rating system needed to be developed that would evaluate and combine reports on the following key questionnaire items: no. 14, results; no. 15, effectiveness ratings; no. 16, meeting expectations; no. 17, adding descriptions of the treatment; no. 18, changes in health, well-being, and adjustment; and no. 19, comparison of ego state therapy with other approaches.

THE RATING SYSTEM

Each client's questionnaire was first "graded" on an alphabetic grading system, much as is often used in college (when grading essay questions). Initially I (JGW) defined the "grades" as follows in terms of effectiveness of the treatment:

A Excellent improvement

B Good (satisfactory) improvement

C Distinctly some, but minimal improvement

D No evidence of improvement

F Negative (perhaps harmful effects) of the treatment

These coincided to some extent with the terms used in item 15, expectations: very effective, somewhat, slightly, ineffective. The checks put in these spaces, however, required considerable modification by the qualitative reports on the other items for the summarized total to emerge in a single letter grade as above. All returns were graded and regraded according to the above until no further changes seemed required.

Next, to objectify these levels further, the preceding criteria were more specifically defined by the rater for each level as follows, and responses graded accordingly:

A 1. Met or exceeded expectations

   2. Results described in superlatives: "excellent," "extraordinary," "outstanding," "powerful"

   3. Rated much higher than (superior to) other therapies experienced

   4. Very significant improvement: loss of symptoms, more successful behavior, greatly improved adjustment, social and otherwise

B 1. Met expectations

   2. Positive recommendation for the therapy

   3. Rated as very good, effective

   4. Significant improvement: symptoms, adjustment, work, living patterns, etc.

C 1. Somewhat (partial) expectations met

   2. Generally favorable attitude toward therapy

   3. Minimal, but positive, results

   4. Evidence of some (but not great) improvement: symptoms, attitudes, living patterns, etc.

D 1. Did not meet expectations; disappointment

   2. Neutral attitude toward therapy

   3. No strongly negative remarks concerning therapy

   4. Very little evidence of improvement: symptoms, attitudes, living patterns

F 1. Distinctly negative results reported; no positive statements; regret at undertaking this therapy

   2. Some indication that symptoms and general adjustment may be worse subsequent to therapy

The questionnaires were carefully re-evaluated (several times until stability was again acquired) and then assigned "effectiveness grades," which are summarized in table 11.

TABLE 11

Summary of Ego State Therapy "Effectiveness" Grade
Assignments on Re-evaluation

GRADE	NO.	% OF TOTAL	
A	23	50%	
B	10	22%	
(A + B)	(33)	(72%)	Considered successful
C	9	19%	Minimally successful
D	4	9%	Considered not successful
F	—	0%	Considered harmful
Total	46	(100%)	

For the resulting grades to be credible, it was important that the ratings be as objective as possible. Accordingly, all questionnaires were read and graded only by one of us (JGW).[8] We did not want the therapist (HHW) to see the questionnaires and perhaps (remembering certain clients from the content) be influenced one way or another.

After reading and reconsidering the grades many different times, it became apparent that even finer gradations were possible. The reported results for some clients were distinctly better than the grade assigned, while others barely met or were slightly less than the stated criteria. These, however, were not sufficient to raise or lower the grade a full step. Accordingly, pluses (+) and minuses (−) were added to the letter grades, resulting in 13 grades being raised to plus and 13 lowered to minus.

In assigning a rating (such as A+ over A) the severity and duration of the referring problem was given consideration. Thus recovery from a lifelong depression or dissociative disorder was given a higher (plus) rating than another case in which the responses to the key items (14, 15, 16, 17, 18, and 19) seemed equally strong, but reported a less severe problem (items 1, 13) or one of much more recent origin (item 2). Similarly so for B, C, and D. Table 12 presents the *final* grades (refined), that is, with adjusted plus or minus signs, and is summarized in table 13.

Note that in table 13 (as contrasted with table 11) I decided to consider grades of C− along with D as "not successful," since the gains were slight and below expectations of either the client or the therapist.

In order that readers can compare ratings with the assigned criteria, repre-

TABLE 12

Final Effectiveness Grades of Individual Therapy Cases

CASE NO.	GRADE	CASE NO.	GRADE
1	C	24	D
2	B	25	A−
3	B−	26	C+
4	D	27	A+
5	A	28	A+
6	A	29	B
7	B−	30	A
8	C−	31	A
9	A+	32	A
10	B−	33	A−
11	A+	34	C−
12	B−	35	A+
13	C	36	A+
14	A−	37	C−
15	D	38	B
16	A+	39	B+
17	A	40	A
18	A−	41	A+
19	A	42	A
20	A−	43	C+
21	C+	44	C
22	B	45	B−
23	D	46	A

sentative cases at each level are now presented with the pertinent data on which the final (refined) rating was based, including the problem, its duration (items 1 and 2) and the type and extent of any prior therapy (items 4 and 5). Comments are quoted directly from the questionnaires.

REPRESENTATIVE CASES AT EACH RATING LEVEL

There were eight *A* + cases. Here are three representative examples.

Case 16

Items 1, 2: Polyfragmented MPD. Lifelong.

TABLE 13

Summary of *Final* Effectiveness Grades for Cases
at Each (Refined) Level

A+	8	
A	10	
A−	5	
B+	2	
B	4	
B−	4	As and Bs = 33 (72%) considered successful
C+	3	
C	3	C+ and C = 6 (13%) minimally successful
C−	3	
D	4	
F	0	C−, D, and F = 7 (15%) not successful*
Total	46	

*Helen pointed out that "not successful" had been assigned only to cases that had been treated in a single "marathon" weekend (8–12 hours) session. It was her position that some of these more difficult cases could have been successfully reached with ego state therapy if there had been more sessions, such as described in chapter 14. Several clients concurred with this point in their questionnaire responses.

Prior therapy

Items 4, 5: Psychoanalytic, cognitive, humanistic. 0–4 per week, 9 years.

Item 7: Somewhat effective.

Item 8: (Expectations met?) Very little.

Ego state therapy

Item 15: Very effective.

Item 16: (Expectations met?) Yes.

Item 17: Amazingly effective treatment. About 70–80% of my healing was accomplished in two weekends.

Item 18: It's been 2 years since I realized that I was fully integrated. I have had no relapses or symptomatic use of defense mechanisms.

Item 19: (Compare with other approaches?) Amazingly effective.

Letter added: Ended abusive marriage. Continued successful career. My life is pretty happy at this point. I am very thankful and grateful to Helen.

Case 28

Items 1, 2: Abuse as a child. Aware of problem a year or so before calling Helen.

Prior therapy

Items 4, 5: Psychoanalytic (3 times a week, 4-1/2 years)

Item 7: Somewhat effective.

Item 8: (Expectations met?) Largely.

Ego state therapy

Item 14: I had dreams, sleep disturbances, crying spells, which all totally disappeared once I had done the therapy.

Item 15: Very effective.

Item 16: (Expectations met?) Yes.

Item 17: I could not have asked for a more successful therapeutic experience. I am extremely satisfied with the results and the speed with which the work was accomplished.

Item 21: (As a therapist have you used ego state therapy?) Yes! And obviously not merely with cases concerning abuse.

Case 35

Items 1, 2: Unresolved dissociative symptoms related to childhood traumas. Sexual issues not fully resolved in 11 years of therapy (age 6).

Prior therapy

Items 4, 5: Psychoanalytic. 2 years in analysis, 9 in psychodynamic therapy.

Item 7: Somewhat effective.

Item 8: (Expectations met?) Partially.

Item 9: It took too long. These therapies were not empowering.

Ego state therapy

Item 15: Very effective.

Item 16: (Expectations met?) Yes.

Item 17: Ego state therapy facilitates access to "places" and "parts" within myself in a real, powerful, experiential way. Helen's presence and support felt more real and available than I've ever experienced.

Item 18: I feel more peace and confident and hopeful as a person and as a therapist. My creativity has increased, and I feel "generative" in more ways than ever. I am more passionate, enthusiastic, and committed to my work as a therapist.

Item 21: (As a therapist have you used ego state therapy?) Yes, with astonishingly positive outcome in relatively *brief* periods of therapy. Clients report feeling *so empowered* to have this new way of working on themselves. I am *committed* to disseminating information to others on this profoundly effective therapy.

There were ten *A* cases. Here are three representative examples.

Case 30

Items 1, 2: Symptoms from childhood molestation—fear of being alone, excessive anxiety, low self-esteem. 25 + years.

Prior therapy

Items 4, 5: Psychoanalytic, cognitive, humanistic, bodywork. 500 hours, 10 years.

Item 6: Symptom improved but still residual fears and feeling of not being integrated.

Item 7: Very effective.

Item 8: (Expectations met?) Yes.

Ego state therapy

Item 11: 3 weekends.

Item 14: Fear went away. Self-esteem and confidence improved markedly. Fear of men greatly decreased. Relationship with husband and mother improved. Much less fear of intimacy.

Item 15: Very effective.

Item 16: (Expectations met?) Yes.

Item 18: I feel internally integrated, whole. Minor asthma symptoms improved.

Item 19: (Compare with other approaches?) It's like speaking directly rather than talking about it. Great relief. Unexpected insight.

Case 32

Items 1, 2: Healing from aftereffects of child abuse. 35–40 years.

Prior therapy

Items 4, 5: Humanistic, hypnotherapy groups (5 + years).

Item 7: Very effective.

Item 8: (Expectations met?) Partially.

Ego state therapy

Item 14: Voice of father transferred into helpful ego state and transformation has been stable. Work of detaching from mother not as complete.

Item 15: Very effective.

Item 16: (Expectations met?) Yes. Exceeded expectations.

Item 17: Idea of positive functioning of destructive ego state is extremely important. It ended my internal civil war.

Item 18: Yes. Seeing you is only part of an ongoing healing. Transformation of internal critic to helpful ego state is probably the greatest gift I got from you.

Case 40

Items 1, 2: Lingering doubts about possible childhood abuse.

Prior therapy

Items 4, 5: Psychoanalytic, cognitive, behavioral. (200 hours, 5 years).

Item 6: Insight better. Still had unresolved issues.

Item 7: Somewhat (effective).

Item 8: (Expectations met?) Partially.

Ego state therapy

Item 14: Uncovered lots of memories, dealt with weight issues, dismissed sexual concerns from childhood.

Item 15: Very effective.

Item 16: (Expectations met?) Yes.

Item 17: I knew I was doing the search, discovering and healing of my problems. It felt safe and like a huge burden was lifted.

Item 18: Lost 25 pounds, still losing—feel more secure.

Item 19: (Compare with other approaches?) Ego state is more intense, rapid, and self-healing.

Item 21: (As a therapist have you used ego state therapy?) Yes, with excellent results. Thanks.

There were five *A* − cases. Here are two representative examples.

Case 14

Items 1, 2: Irrational overreaction, anger, anxiety, insecurity.

Prior therapy

Items 4, 5: Sullivanian, cognitive, systemic (250 hours, 2–3 years).

Item 7: Somewhat (effective).

Item 8: (Expectations met?) Largely.

Ego state therapy

Item 14: Much calmer sense of self; fewer overreactions; inaccurate conclusions re: self corrected. Accessed or activated a wiser facet of self (observing ego).

Item 15: Very effective.

Item 16: (Expectations met?) Yes.

Item 17: Helen's guided imagery was incredibly intuitive; she's a natural healer.

Item 18: Calmer, more centered, less reactive, increased self confidence.

Item 19: (Compare with other approaches?) Similar to Gestalt approach, integrating various facets of psyche.

Added letter: Thank you again. The benefits of my work with you have been dramatic and long-lasting.

Case 18

Items 1, 2: Resolution of childhood trauma. Explore relationships. 1 year that I was firsthand aware of.

Prior therapy

Items 4, 5: Humanistic. 6–8 hours (2 months).

Item 6: Negligible (results).

Item 7: Ineffective.

Item 8: (Expectations met?) Very little.

Ego state therapy

Item 14: I left the weekend feeling lighter (relieved) and like a worthwhile, lovable person.

Item 15: Very effective.

Item 16: (Expectations met?) Yes.

Item 17: The issue I planned to address in therapy became secondary; to my surprise, issues surrounding my mother emerged and were resolved—whew!

Item 18: Yes. My well-being has improved. My relationships with men have changed. I'm now making more responsible choices.

There was 1 *B+* case. Here it is.

Case 39

Items 1, 2: Depression. 6 months.

Prior therapy

Items 4, 5: Psychoanalytic (once a week, 2 years), humanistic (10 years).

Item 6: Basically good (results).

Item 7: Somewhat (effective).

Item 8: (Expectations met?) Partially.

Ego state therapy

Item 15: Very effective. Good for the goals I had at the time.

Item 16: (Expectations met?) Yes.

Item 17: I had worked with ego states before, but this therapy uncovered states that were amnesic to me.

Item 18: I feel freer of old habitual patterns of self-critical thinking.

Item 19: (Compare with other approaches?) Similar to work I did with an expert on dissociative and PTSD states. Your work more complete.

There were four *B* cases. Here are two representative examples.

Case 2

Items 1, 2: Resolve childhood traumas affecting current relationships. 45 years.

Prior therapy

Items 4, 5: Psychoanalytic (10 years), humanistic, hypnotherapy.

Item 7: Very effective.

Item 8: (Expectations met?) Largely.

Item 9: (Refers to ego state therapy as "hypnotherapy.") The ease of resolutions was quite different from the gain in long-term analysis. The quickness of change.

Ego state therapy

Item 14: I felt understood, not shamed.

Item 15: Very effective.

Item 16: (Expectations met?) Yes.

Item 17: The dreams afterward were quite important. I felt more sensitive and able to interpret my unconscious processes after therapy.

Item 18: Felt happier. I could connect states which were at odds with my beliefs better. My feelings didn't override my good sense.

Item 19: (Compare with other approaches?) Was in Bio E, which was too painful. Interview analysis with Perlian was too slow and focused on affect and no debriefing in the process, which was essential in ego-state integration.

Case 29

Items 1, 2: Guilt, history of drug abuse, sexual acting-out. Since age 22.

Prior therapy

Items 4, 5: Psychoanalytic (3–4 years).

Item 6: No behavioral change.

Item 7: Somewhat effective.

Item 8: (Expectations met?) Partially.

Ego state therapy

Item 14: I have experienced a reduction in self-criticism and guilt feelings with acceptance of self.

Item 15: Very effective.

Item 16: (Expectations met?) Yes.

Item 19: Remarried. Major career change. Good health.

Item 21: Many thanks for your help.

There were four *B−* cases. Here are two representative examples.

Case 7

Items 1, 2: Mid-life depression, relationship failures, low self-esteem. Lifelong.

Prior therapy

Items 4, 5: Cognitive, behavioral, hypnotherapy (3 years, 20 years ago).

Item 6: Unfinished business. Uneasiness.

Item 7: Very effective.

Item 8: (Expectations met?) Largely.

Item 9: Cognitive therapy was good. Ended disastrously.

Ego state therapy

Item 15: Somewhat (effective).

Item 16: (Expectations met?) Largely.

Item 17: I have always wondered if I was recalling dreams/daydreams whatever. I seem to have unclogged something.

Item 18: Better adjusted. Powerful. Husband can't absorb my personality. Less the victim.

Item 19: (Compare with other approaches?) Talking helped form a personal image, emotional history, which has a good value. It couldn't crack "the nut." (Client is referring to prior cognitive therapy.)

Case 12

Items 1, 2: Depression (duration unanswered).

Prior therapy

Items 4, 5: Psychoanalytic, humanistic (150 hours, 2-1/2 years).

Item 7: Somewhat effective.

Item 8: (Expectations met?) Largely.

Ego state therapy

Item 14: Moderately helpful.

Item 15: Somewhat effective.

Item 16: (Expectations met?) Partially.

Item 17: Not enough time. I'm pretty well defended.

Item 18: Continuous improvement.

Item 19: (Compare with other approaches?) In right circumstances, nothing can touch it.

There were 3 *C+* cases. Here is one representative example.

Case 43

Items 1, 2: Depression and anxiety (since adolescence).

Prior therapy

Items 4, 5: Psychoanalytic (5 years).

Item 7: Somewhat effective.

Item 8: (Expectations met?) Partially.

Ego state therapy

Item 14: Managed the "pain" most of the time.

Item 15: Somewhat effective.

Item 16: (Expectations met?) Largely.

Item 17: Did not achieve the breakthrough I had anticipated and wanted. This may be unrealistic.

Item 18: Having worked on the problems minimized their roles and potency in my life; accept that they are part of me.

There were three *C* cases. Here is one representative example.

Case 1

Items 1, 2: Frequent experiences of sinking self-esteem. Forever.

Prior therapy

Items 4, 5: Psychoanalytic (20 years).

Item 7: Somewhat effective.

Item 8: (Expectations met?) Partially.

Ego state therapy

Item 14: Think I understand better the origins of my self-rejection and self-criticism and self-defeating behavior.

Item 15: Somewhat effective.

Item 16: (Expectations met?) Partially.

Item 17: I had difficulty going into deep trance.

Item 18: Continue to grow in awareness, but also continue to be self-rejecting and at times self-defeating.

Item 19: (Compare with other approaches?) The experience of altered states has opportunity for deeper exploration of memory.

There were three C− cases. Here is one typical example.

Case 8

Items 1, 2: Depression. Several years.

Prior therapy

Items 4, 5: Psychoanalytic, humanistic (100 hours, 2 years).

Item 6: (Results) Modest help.

Item 7: Somewhat effective.

Item 8: (Expectations met?) Partially.

Ego state therapy

Item 14: (Results) Modest.

Item 15: Slightly effective.

Item 16: (Expectations met?) Partially.

Item 18: (Changes since therapy?) Not anything significant.

Item 19: (Compare with other approaches?) Yes. With L.S. Barkdale approach, which I found best for me.

There were four *D* cases. Here are two representative examples.

Case 4

Items 1, 2: Infertility, marital discord, depression. 2-1/2 years.

Prior therapy

Items 4, 5: Cognitive (2-1/2 years, once weekly).

Item 7: Somewhat effective.

Item 8: (Expectations met?) Partially.

Ego state therapy

Item 14: (No answer).

Item 15: Somewhat effective.

Item 16: (Expectations met?) Partially.

Item 18: (Changes since therapy?) Not really.

Case 23

Items 1, 2: (No answer).

Items 4, 5: No prior psychotherapy.

Item 14: (No answer).

Item 15: Slightly effective.

Item 16: (Expectations met?) Very Little.

Item 18: (Changes since therapy?) "No."

Before summarizing the questionnaire results, it is of interest to consider the responses to item 17. It called for a completely unstructured comment. The respondents were simply asked to "Add anything you wish to describe it" (that is, their ego state therapy experience). The contrast between the 8 A+ (most successful) cases and the seven C− and D (not successful) cases was quite revealing.

Responses to Item 17 (Add Anything You Wish)

A+ Cases

9: It was incredible.

11: Interestingly, I remember very few of the details of the work, who the ego states are, and what they believe and feel.

16: Amazingly effective treatment. About 70–80% of my healing was accomplished in two weekends.

27: Every therapist should be exposed to this way of working–whether they think they're going to use it or not.

28: I could not have asked for a more successful therapeutic experience. I am extremely satisfied with the results and the speed with which the work was accomplished.

35: Ego state therapy facilitates access to 'places' and 'parts' within myself in a real, powerful, experiential way. Helen's presence and support felt more real and available than I've ever experienced.

36: Helen Watkins, a loving, acutely present practitioner who totally focuses with the moment–a gifted healer.[9]

41: Please see attached note. Note: There is a sustaining quality about ego state work which has followed me (supported me) down through the years. Put me back into the center of my own world– in charge and responsible for it. Ego state work is the most effective approach I've seen yet.

C– and D cases

4: (No response)

8: (No response)

15: (No response)

23: (No response)

24: Benign.

34: Given the intensity of my defenses, I needed many more hours and also greater depth of trance. What impacted me most was the compassion and empathy and initiative Helen deployed.

37: (No response)

Summary

The results of this follow-up study might be summarized as follows:

1. 46 clients out of a total of 86 (53%) returned the questionnaires– anonymously, as desired.

2. Considering the amount of time involved since their treatment sessions with HHW, (3 months to 17 years, median 2 years), this percent of return compares most favorably with those typically secured in other research studies covering an equally lengthy period.

3. The reasons for entering therapy (problems) covered a wide range of neurotic, psychosomatic, and behavioral disorders, most frequent of which were: depression, childhood traumas, low self-esteem, anxiety, marital and sexual problems, dissociation, performance anxiety, compulsions, and addictions (in order of most to least frequent).

4. Their durations were as follows:

"Lifelong," 20 years or greater	$N = 23$ (50%)
"Intermediate," 2 to 19 years	$N = 15$ (33%)
"Recent," less than 2 years	$N = 3$ (07%)
"Misc.," training, no real problem	$N = 5$ (10%)

5. Thirty three (72%) of all questionnaires returned were rated from A+ to B−, and considered as *successful*.

6. Six (13%) of all questionnaires returned were rated C+ or C, and considered as having *minimal success*.

7. Seven (15%) of all questionnaires returned, were rated C−, D, or F and considered as *not successful*.

8. Ego state therapy was given significantly higher ratings in effectiveness ($p < .005$) when compared by all respondents ($N = 46$) to other approaches in which they had prior treatment experiences.

9. Ego state therapy was rated significantly higher than prior therapies ($p < .005$) in meeting expectations, and given a "yes" more than three times as often (26 : 8).

10. Specifically, ego state therapy was given significantly higher ratings in effectiveness ($p < .005$) than psychoanalytic therapy by those who had experienced both ($N = 27$).

11. Clients rated ego state therapy significantly higher than prior psychoanalytic therapy ($p < .005$) in meeting their expectations.

12. As to ego state therapy's *relative* efficiency, many clients commented on the speed, an 8–15-hour weekend (median $= 11$ hours), as compared to their prior therapies (range: 10 to 500+ hours, median 145, over 2 months to 38 years).

13. Those with prior psychoanalytic therapy ($N = 27$) reported a range of 18 to 500+ hours, median 150, over 2 months to 38 years, median 5 years. Seven respondents reported their prior psychoanalytic therapy as having a frequency of from 1 to 5 sessions per week, median 3.

The question remains as to whether the 42 clients (47%) who did not return the questionnaire would have been rated similarly to the 46 respondents. One can only guess that many reasons, such as wrong address, lack of interest in responding, unsuccessful treatment, and deceased, might be factors.

One also cannot say as to what part of its treatment effect can be attributed to ego state theory, what part to ego state techniques, what part to the use of clinical hypnosis, what part to the intensive "marathon" weekend format, what to the selectivity of the population, or what to the experience and skill of the therapist. Nor can one generalize its efficiency when applied in a different format (e.g., one hour a week) by other therapists.

However, we have received enthusiastic communications from numerous colleagues who have applied this approach to their own patients. Many of them have added to and developed further, both ego state theory and ego state techniques (see Edelstein, 1982; Frederick, 1993, 1994, 1996; Frederick & McNeal, 1993; Frederick & Phillips, 1995; Gainer & Torem, 1993; Hartman, 1995; Phillips, 1993; Torem, 1993).

SELECTIVITY OF THE POPULATION

The majority of the clients were active mental health professionals who had already been informed about ego state therapy through workshops and the reading of publications. They would not have gone to the expense of flying to Montana for personal "marathon" weekend treatment unless they were already highly motivated and anticipating results.

On the other hand, since so many were practicing therapists themselves, who had experienced prior sessions of personal treatment, they were in a good position to evaluate the relative effectiveness of their ego state therapy.

A CONTROLLED EXPERIMENTAL STUDY

A recent clinical-experimental study on the effectiveness of ego state therapy in the treatment of migraine has been conducted at the Shealy Institute in Springfield, Missouri, in association with Victoria University in Melbourne, Australia (Emmerson & Farmer, 1996). They report the effect of 4 sessions of ego state therapy on 10 "menstrual migraine" sufferers.

Subjects were administered the MMPI-2 and the Beck Depression Inventory, pre- and post-treatment. A time series design revealed that the average number of days of headaches per month declined significantly from 12.2 to 2.95 ($p < .05$). Significant changes in the MMPI-2 on "depression, anger and extroversion" were reported, as were significant changes on the Beck Depression Inventory.

We hope colleagues, therapists and researchers, will undertake more such controlled studies, and on other clinical populations.

We believe that many practitioners, especially those who are trained in, and practice psychodynamic therapies, will find the ego state approach meets today's demands of managed care and other third-party payers for a brief therapy that is both effective and efficient, and that can produce permanent, constructive change—not mere symptom relief—in patients with psychological problems.

14

THE PROTECTOR DEFENDS HIS FORTRESS: A DIFFICULT, COMPLEX CASE

Wilhelm Reich (1949) contributed to psychoanalysis the concepts of "character armor" and "character analysis." He noted that many extremely difficult cases were resistant to usual psychoanalytic treatment because their "resistances" were frozen into a rigid, protective armor designed to protect the ego from inner and outer threats. This armor manifested much more continuous and severe resistances than are exhibited in normal defense processes. It fiercely wards off the therapeutic goal of insight, which would upset its equilibrium.

According to Reich, this character armor must be aggressively analyzed before normal resistances and defense maneuvers can be attacked. In this armor, enormous quantities of basic affects (sexuality and anxiety) are repressed. To these two Reich added a third, anger or hatred, noting that when we talk about "boiling inside," we are referring to undischarged anger or hatred.

In the very difficult, stubborn, and relatively untreatable cases, this inner rage is so strong that the ego dares not let go of it. Character analysis required the systematic working-through of various levels of development with the expectation that these rigid character resistances in the armor would rise time and again in the treatment. Accordingly, successful psychoanalytic treatment of such patients often required hundreds of hours over many years.

Therapy of such cases was very lengthy because of the threat that penetrating the armor too rapidly might cause a flooding of rage into the ego with violent suicidal or homicidal acting-out by the patient.

The case of Mary, which Helen (HHW) describes here, represents just such a patient. Her character armor, termed "the Fortress" was stoutly defended by an ego state, who came to be known as "the Protector."

The treatment was very difficult, very complex, very hazardous, and much longer than the ego state cases described in chapters 11 and 13. However, it was undertaken in the more traditional once-a-week format. Such a case, requiring therapist relationship availability, and even possible hospitalization, could not (and should not) be undertaken in a single weekend marathon.

Mary was brought to me by a roommate, who caught her holding a gun to her head, ready to pull the trigger. Thus began a three-year tortuous path to healing, a path fraught with mutilation and the ever-present cloud of suicide. A few years earlier she had been hospitalized in another state on two occasions for suicide attempts using medications.

She was not afraid of death. She was afraid of life. She wanted to feel emotion like other human beings she encountered, but could not. She could not even feel pain when she cut herself. Her willingness to see me was her last hope in finding life, and she made it clear this would be her last effort. She also made it abundantly clear she would commit suicide if hospitalized. I knew she was serious and determined to carry out her decision. The only reason she agreed to see me was because she learned I used hypnosis, which she had never experienced before.

I agreed to treat her only if she would be willing to see a psychiatrist for medication. That she did, but after a few months it was evident that the Prozac he prescribed had little effect on her. Other medications from the previous hospitalizations also had little value in changing her mental state, according to the patient.

Thus we began our journey—she with much doubt, I with much trepidation.

This case of ego state therapy required time, time to develop trust, not only with the waking patient, but particularly with states only available through hypnosis.

At the first appointment my impression of her was that of an impenetrable fortress. Her somewhat heavy but strong body slowly eased into the client chair. Her energy felt weighty, almost palpable, as if it had solidity. The expression on her face was serious, dour, and distant, barely in contact with me. I hardly knew where to begin, so I listened.

In measured tones she gave a partial history as if painting a canvas with disconnected blotches. In reality she was a part-time college senior in art and a part-time employee in a local store. Being in her early thirties, she was older than most of her fellow students and more experienced. Reticent to speak, she made few friends on or off campus.

She had few memories before age 10, when her parents divorced. Father had been a hell's-fire-and-damnation type of minister but left the ministry to seek his fortunes in business. She knew she had been deathly afraid of him but not sure why. She recalled her mother being hysterical after the divorce and so unpredictable that Mary had to care for her two much-younger brothers, ages 2 and 4. She also remembered being so angry at about age 6 that she threw some kittens against a wall so hard that they died. At age 5 she was bitten in the face by a dog, but there was no plastic surgery until age 18, when she paid for it herself. She used street drugs from age 13 to 20 but none since then. A persistent thought in her head declared: "If I'm not perfect, I should be dead."

The first session produced these disjointed snatches of memory, very suggestive of an unhappy childhood within a dysfunctional family. My first goal was to develop our relationship by carefully listening and resonating and to build ego strength within her, if possible. With her eyes closed and no attempt at a hypnotic induction, I taught her my safe room technique (see chapter 10), including the perceived core of strength, which she pictured as a fluffy white dog. She recalled as a young child she had a stuffed white animal that she cuddled. In addition, I gave her my *Raising Self-Esteem* tape (Watkins, H., 1990a) to play before sleep. This was not a time to interrogate or to probe with hypnosis. Rather, it was a time for gradually building trust. And it was a time for constructive psychological homework that would give her hope.

I told her I needed something from her, a written statement to stop her from a suicide attempt. After some discussion she finally wrote the following: "I will stay alive. If I feel that I cannot stay alive, I will get a friend to take me to the Health Service, where they can protect me from myself."

Since she was a very conscientious and successful undergraduate student, I assumed she would abide by her statement, at least consciously, even though unconscious motivations might differ. It also set the stage for the idea that not all behaviors were okay with me, that there were boundaries to be considered.

Each session, depending upon what we touched upon, ended with an assignment of psychological homework, which she followed faithfully. She had learned early in life to do what she was told and to do it perfectly. Since perfection is impossible, the effort was doomed to failure, not only from the criticism she received from her parents, but also in her mind. Thus I had an opportunity to laud her for any effort that she made, regardless of result. Therefore, through a subtle way, in our relationship I hoped she might learn that she is neither bad nor deserves to die if she is not perfect. Simply telling her that the attempt to be perfect is foolish would have been fruitless. Besides, it would have reinforced her idea that she was wrong and therefore bad.

Furthermore, the homework each week gave her a focus of activity from which she could derive hope for potential healing and a feeling that she could do something to help herself. Without any psychological effort on her part, she could easily fall back to her depressive thoughts and behavior. If she simply waited to see me each week, she might come to believe that I could do it for her, which would certainly lead to disillusionment, hopelessness, and perhaps even suicide.

Homework at first consisted of simple cognitive assignments, such as trying to change "shoulds" to "wants" in her thinking and behavior, with the intention of eroding some of her unreasonable feelings of guilt. Also, it would reinforce the idea that it is permissible for her to "want," an idea foreign to her since she had been taught to do the bidding of others.

When telling me about her feelings in childhood, the homework changed to simple imagery. For example, she was able to tell me of her anger at mother, but as soon as I asked her to express those feelings to mother in a chair, she froze. In other words, she could tell me about feelings but could not express them. She recalled feeling both angry and guilty at age 10 when her mother made her take care of the younger brothers—angry at the responsibility and guilty because "I didn't know enough." The homework for this session was to close her eyes and visualize that 10-year-old and nurture her in some way. She needed to begin to learn compassion and understanding for her own internal self.

As we progressed, more memories began to emerge. She recalled a 5-year-old experience when mother was in bed, pregnant, and yelling at her to do the washing. When Mary protested, mother screamed, "Do you want the baby to die?" When mother complained to father, father hit Mary. She also remembered crying when the parents had her puppy killed for biting a neighbor child who teased it. Father hit her to stop crying. The rules were clear: Don't cry, don't feel, don't complain, do what you are told, and do it right even if you don't know how.

During the above session I attempted a hand levitation induction, but there was no movement. I continued the induction via relaxing visualization to have her view the 5-year-old and nurture it in any way she could. There were no words, but finger signals indicated she could see the child and try to help it.

The purpose of beginning the hypnotic induction was to touch upon unconscious dimensions, thus deepening the therapeutic process. I was well aware of the psychological fortress she had built, no doubt for good reason. That fortress must contain powerful forces. Otherwise, why bother to build it? I knew I must be careful not to try to break it down with a frontal assault but rather to penetrate a niche here and there that would not be too threatening to its contents.

By the third month of our therapy I decided it was time to release some of her anger physically. I asked her to choose some physical task that might express anger. She chose to chop up an old couch ready for the dumpster. That felt good. She could justify the task as work that needed to be done.

Subsequently I taught her my silent abreaction technique (see chapter 9), which she could practice at home when she wished. That technique brought about an internal reaction. She told me she was aware of a Censor inside (whom she pictured as a TV preacher in black), who determined what she could say or do. "The Censor gives me the idea that I can feel anything I want as long as I please the world on the outside and not reveal my emotions." Here was the internal replication of the admonitions of her parents. She also said the Censor was getting upset at her for revealing her emotions to me. I explained that this Censor was trying to protect her in the only way he knew how, but that his internal behavior was destructive to Mary.

An attempted hand levitation induction again produced no movement, but I spoke as if speaking directly to the Censor, reiterating the above protective motivation and the resultant damage to Mary. It was my first attempt at knocking on the door of the fortress, and my first attempt at trying to make friends with whatever was inside.

Mary was still playing the *Self-Esteem* tape but noticed the fantasy room had become empty of furniture and therefore not relaxing or inviting. Something or someone (the Censor?) was interfering with this positive imagery. I urged her to talk to the Censor with understanding of his motivation and to treat the child with caring when recalling events of the past.

Since movement in a hand levitation induction could easily be thwarted by unconscious processes, I began using H. Spiegel's "eye roll" (1973). That technique evidences hypnotic ability by the amount of white showing upon eye closure. I used this procedure to ask the "unconscious mind" to take her to some significant experience out of the past. Finger signals indicated no. It was clear I was alerting the contents of the fortress.

I decided it was time for me to be more active. She recalled at the age of 6 coming into her grandparents' house with a hurt knee. Her uncle, age 12, kicked her other leg and said, "Now you won't think about your knee." Under hypnosis I regressed her to that scene. She was too afraid to say anything. Therefore, with her permission, I stepped into the scene, ordered the uncle out of the house and confronted the grandparents for not protecting her.

Thus far I had upset the forces inside the fortress. I must not now step back in fear, but instead let them know I was someone to be reckoned with. More important, those forces needed to learn that I was an ally, not an enemy, by rescuing the little girl of the past. Sweet words and gentleness would suggest weakness and produce derision. My method of protecting would be different, but my motivation would be the same—protection. Our struggle would be on our differing methods of protecting.

My rescuing behavior would have seemed silly at the cognitive, waking level, but we were dealing with hypnotic or unconscious processes. Trance logic is quite different. The past becomes real, as if happening in the present. The thinking is simple and concrete, like that of a child.

In the following session she felt worse. She had cut herself to relieve the emotional pain. (Her cutting had never required hospitalization.) She did not feel the physical pain of cutting, but the cutting relieved the unbearable emotional pain. I had become a threat to the contents of the fortress. She heard the Censor tell her that he had cut her to stop feeling and not to see me anymore, but Mary and I had formed a trusting relationship and she had no intention of leaving therapy.

In the hope of finding more benevolent behaviors to substitute for her cutting, I hypnotized her and simply asked the "inner mind" through finger signaling to give her suggestions for relieving emotional pain. The purpose of the cutting was to stop emotional pain, but more generally to stop feeling altogether. With no definite response from the fingers, I wondered out loud if she could express feelings indirectly through exercise, freestyle art drawing, doodles, or finger painting. The finger signals agreed. The finger signals also agreed to tell Mary that the things that happened in her childhood were not her fault—a most important idea for her to absorb.

After the cutting incident, I concluded that the Censor might be willing to talk to me directly under hypnosis. "What do you want to know?" was the curt response. "How old was Mary when you came to be?" I wanted to understand his origin.

"She was 3; time for her to grow up. She was at a friend's house with her parents there. Her girlfriend jumped off a dresser and broke an arm. Parents blamed Mary and punished her. That's when I came to be." (Actually his very beginning may have been at the first trauma a few months earlier, mentioned later in this chapter, but he may not have taken full form until the above incident.)

We talked about his caring, protective function, for which I showed my admiration. However, he made it clear he did not love her, because "love is dangerous." When those who are supposed to love you, abuse you instead, then certainly love must seem dangerous.

It was important to have direct contact with the keeper of the fortress—an ego state who had power and directed her life from within.

Now that the Censor and I had become directly acquainted, I decided to start abreactive work but with safe distancing. Under hypnosis I established a scene where Mary and I were sitting on one side of a glass wall observing "a woman who looks like you becoming younger and younger until she becomes a little girl, then tell me what happens." (In this method the patient takes me wherever she is ready to go.) She saw herself at age 6 going to the barn with her 12-year-old uncle who grabs her and orders her to take her clothes off. Mary turned away from the scene because "it's too painful to watch." I told her, "That's fine, but you can say or do anything you want to the uncle." After about a minute of silence she informed me she killed him, rescued the little girl and brought her to where we were sitting. However, the little girl, she said, was still frightened because she didn't trust anyone.

The principle of standing up to the abuser in fantasy (not reality) is an essential aspect of abreactive therapy. The abused patient must get his or her power back, most easily accomplished through regression in hypnosis. When working with trauma from the past, the problem remains in the patient's head as it was experienced and implanted then, and it is there internally where under regression it must be re-experienced. Simply confronting the abuser of the past in the reality of the present does not alter that implantation, and it often creates new reality problems for the patient – personal, family, and legal.

The above abreaction was very mild in form, but it was a beginning in the right direction toward healing. I wondered if there would be any reaction from the Censor.

Apparently there was none, as the week went smoothly. At the following session she recalled that at age 5 she broke her collarbone in a fall, but her parents would not believe she was badly hurt. Mother called her a wimp, and father hit her for crying. Under hypnosis I again established the room with the window wall observing "a woman who looks like you getting younger and younger until she reaches age 5." Unlike the previous abreaction (which was *watching*) now she becomes age 5 and *experiences* the scene of falling against a piano bench, breaking her collarbone (years later corroborated by x-ray) and crying.[1] Mother derides her for crying and father hits her to stop crying, "but I can't stop because it hurts too much." This time she can't confront the abusers because "I am not allowed to" and "they wouldn't listen anyway."

It is interesting to note that she could confront a lesser abuser, the uncle, but not the parents. Since she viewed the Censor as a minister in black, I assumed that he was the introjection of father. Therefore the Censor would internally direct her to follow father's rules, such as "Don't cry, don't feel, be perfect, be obedient," with a rigidity that must have come from the original source.

During the next several sessions she talked about her anger at her parents. She beat a pillow when she couldn't sleep one night, spitefully using her left hand. "I was naturally left-handed but they changed me to the right hand because writing with the left hand was evil." Such expressions were useful in understanding her own feelings about her parents, but they were only words. There was very little release of affect. Perhaps a few puffs of smoke from the fortress, but that's about all.

I searched for different avenues of approach. My Door of Forgiveness technique (chapter 10) was ineffective, because she refused to go through any of the doors, plaintively saying "feelings hurt too much." I switched the scene to a Wise One on top of a mountain, having her ask whatever she wished. In silence she asked the anger to be taken away. The Wise One told her it could do so but that it would not help her in the long run (truly wise advice). Then I asked her to go back to a time when she believed in Jesus and to talk to Him silently. She reported that Christ told her that lots of people hurt him but that didn't mean He was bad, and that He was angry too when He threw the money changers out of the temple.

This source of authority had internal meaning. If the Censor was an intro-jection of father when Mary was a child, then the Censor would actually be a child state and subject to child thinking. The idea that one might not be bad if others are abusive and the concept that anger could be justified probably seeped into the fortress. These ideas had impact.

I continued abreactions by asking the "inner mind" to take her where she needed to go. The scenes dealt with father, who was physically, sexually, and emotionally abusive. Sometimes I brought in Jesus to help her. Then she would tell me what He did, such as, "He put a bandage on my knee." At other times the adult-hypnotized Mary agreed to rescue the little girl in the scene and tell her it was not her fault, that she was not bad. I wanted to reinforce the concept of innocence and the justification of anger.

She was finally able to use the silent abreaction and make positive self-statements in that technique, such as, "I'm smart."

During one session I asked the "inner mind" to take her where she needed to go to discharge more anger. "I'm in the hospital visiting Daddy who has the mumps. Mommy told me it was my fault because I gave it to him. So I put my hand in the fan to hurt myself to show I'm sorry." In another session she kicked some kittens because "they loved me so I had to hurt them." The day before the molestation by the uncle, he told her he loved her. The day after the molestation she burned herself. Here were the beginnings of self-mutilation.

These were times of struggles and resistance to learn about her childhood innocence. It seemed as if she were programmed from day one that she was bad. To her, love equaled pain, and pain equaled forgiveness. "Only bad people feel bad; good people don't." She had sleepless nights, agitated depres-sion, confusion. She felt suicidal. Sometimes she spent the night at the

Health Service to feel safe. Only when too anxiety-ridden did she cut herself. Occasionally she was able to cry. We dealt with the interpretation of dreams, some of which seemed like re-experiencing traumas. I continued to ask the "inner mind" to take her where she needed to go to progress healing. I trusted her unconscious to be the safest and best guide in therapy, because it would not overwhelm her with more than she could handle. The rigid thinking of the past was unrelenting. "Even if you think anger, you are evil." The frustration to release anger, and the prohibition against it escalated. I constantly defended her righteous anger. I intervened in some scenes, or had her rescue the child. The "inner mind" helped most often in the rescuing to take the abused child to a safe place. We struggled together.

It was evident that the "inner mind" had form, was able to act, had wisdom, and was benevolent. It was an ego state, which Mary named the Higher Self. Months later we graduated from finger signals to speech, which made communication much easier.

I asked the Higher Self to take her to the first time she shut off anger. She became age 2, entered her house to get a drink of water. Father told her to shut the door. She said no because she was just getting a quick drink. He became enraged and almost beat her to death. She decided never to cry or feel again to stop the pain of the beating. Thereafter she remained still when father abused her. This incident was the beginning of dissociation.

After the 2-year-old abreaction she sometimes felt the pain of the beating in her body as a somatic memory. This scene was the most difficult to process. So much fear, so much anguish, so much pain. She was afraid to face the fantasized father for fear of retribution, also true of scenes in which she was older. The Higher Self helped her express anger in her dreams, which, it said, would relieve tension and be less stressful. This abreaction required many repetitions to work through. It was the most important because it represented the origin of the fractionation. Finally the 2-year-old child could be rescued into a safe environment—a room of her own, playing with a puppy.

She was looking for something terrible that she might have done wrong to justify father's brutality. "If he punished me for nothing, then it's too painful to face that no one loved me."

Here is the most difficult realization to accept for any human being—not to be loved by one's parents or early caregivers. If the fountain from which I spring rejects me, then I am nothing. I don't deserve to exist. Birth was an error, and death is justified.

However, the Higher Self and I were fighting for the rightness of her birth and the wrongness of her parents, whom I simply described as being sick and unable to love her. I emphasized that their inability to love did not mean that she was not lovable.

Who did love this child? Except for uninvolved grandparents, there was no adult in her life except an aunt who lived in a nearby state, and whom she saw on rare visits. The aunt would hold her and gently talk to her. Even if she didn't believe she deserved such attention, it gave her hope.

The inside of the fortress was clearly in an uproar. Eventually, however, the fortress must fall because all the self-knowledge contained therein was false.

By now a year had passed, and despite all the pain, she was still alive and functioning well in her life. In fact, she was able to cry with her roommate and tell her of her childhood—a very first revealing of her history and feelings to anyone except me. Much to her surprise, her roommate did not reject her. Instead of silence and retreat, Mary became self-assertive when offended. Aside from abreactive work, we also processed our hypnotic work, her relationships with others, and with me. It was a global effort to encompass all phases of her life. But we were far from finished. The fortress was damaged but still intact.

Assuming that the Censor was behind the resistance, I spoke with him again. In the meantime Mary decided to call him the Protector, a designation he liked. He had become more malleable, but still adamant about excessive feeling. "I won't cut her if she doesn't feel too much." Obviously the Protector did the cutting. With the gradual breaking down of his resistance, he became more confused. He didn't know what the new rules were supposed to be, so he held on tighter to the old ones. He was certain if he let her feel, she would be destroyed. Black and white rules he could understand, but grays were intolerable.

I was reminded of the logic of a similar protective state in another patient, created during a severe abuse experience. "I have to hurt her, or the world will hurt her more." At the moment of trauma, a created state knows nothing except the experience of the trauma.

During the second year of therapy, the emphasis shifted slightly away from abreactive therapy to concentrating on the relationship between ego states. Significantly, she began to draw scenes of the abuse, which had been prohibited internally because it was a way of revealing the past. Often she had been told by threat of death by her father not to tell, and she never told anyone as she grew up, not even her mother. However, during a present phone call from her mother, living in another state, mother remembered the 2-year-old incident. "I couldn't stand to see you hurt, and I was afraid of your father, so I walked out of the house." That phone call confirmed mother's inadequacy and lack of protectiveness.

In one drawing (see figure 3) she drew the Protector holding in the feelings of fear and anger in a tightened circle. I empathized with the Protector at the burden of holding in so much affect. During one session Mary complained of

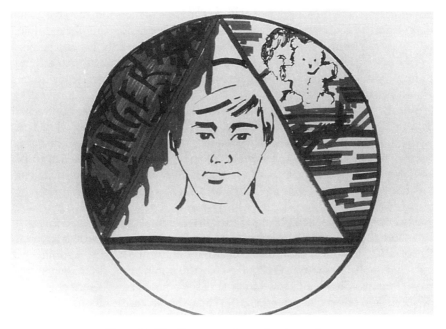

Figure 3. The Protector, drawn by the patient.

anger tension within her, feeling that she might explode. I conferred with the Higher Self to ask if he could do anything to titrate the anger. We discussed the picture of the Protector that she had drawn. I wondered if he could work out something mechanical that would relieve some of that anger energy. The following session Mary brought in a diagram of a fuse box connected to the picture of the Protector, with resistors, a circuit breaker and a switch to reduce and control affect. With the consent of the Protector, the fuse box went into operation and stayed until it no longer was needed, near the end of therapy. (I am always amazed at the ingenious resources inside the human being.)

With the help of the Higher Self the 2-year-old girl was now residing in a room at the end of a hallway, and the Protector became willing to stay in another room nearby. Now it was easier to communicate with each one. During most sessions Mary and I would walk down the stairs in hypnosis. I would visit each room and do whatever needed to be done psychologically. Ironically, at first they were hesitant about the hypnotized adult Mary coming into their room, because they didn't know her. I had been developing a relationship with each of them in the abreactive work. The hypnotized Mary was not separately involved when they were re-experiencing the past. The dissociation became very clear. The child would experience pain, for example, but Mary would not feel it in the waking state or vice versa. For integration to take place, they needed to get acquainted and to give some of their feelings to her. My function must become less important, so that dependency on me would lessen.

During the second, year I worked with the hypnotized Mary, the Higher Self, the Protector, and the Little Girl ego state. In order to bring wholeness to the disparate parts, it was still necessary to return to the original splitting at age 2. The emotional feelings needed to be expressed, the abuser had to be confronted, the bodily feelings had to be felt. We were far from finished. The Protector wavered but was still wary of my procedure. It became clear he feared for his lack of purpose if all his power were taken away. No ego state wants to disappear. The fight for life is universal in all living things. Reassurance and looking at options for protecting were cooly regarded by him. During one hypnotic session the Protector didn't want Mary in his room, but he asked me to come in. "Tell Mary to stop yammering about giving her more feelings. She wants too much and she's not ready." Overprotective, perhaps, but protective nonetheless. When the Protector cut her "because she was hurting from crying," the hypnotized Mary accused him of trying to protect himself from the pain of the tears. Very astute.

The Protector also displayed other vulnerabilities. He couldn't bear to hurt the Little Girl, so he asked me to tell her why her Daddy didn't love her. I did so, explaining father's inability to love, and also taught her that "Daddy had bad anger, but the Protector has good anger." That message was well received and important because at that time she was afraid of the Protector.

With each abreaction at age 2, I asked the Protector and the Little Girl separately to give Mary at least some of the pain they held. When they did that, the hypnotized Mary thanked each for their efforts. They needed to learn that neither Mary nor the system would disintegrate in this process. Obviously it was hard on the unhypnotized Mary, but somehow she managed to function in the world despite the gradual unleashing of this emotional trauma. After each repetition, the internal ego states felt better, but Mary felt worse. No wonder. Sometimes she felt suicidal. Sometimes she wondered if therapy was worth the pain. But having started down this road, there was no turning back. To do so might be more damaging than never to have started at all. Half-finished would leave her in a state of constant turmoil. There was no way to reconstruct the fortress. Her stated goal at the beginning of therapy was to *feel*, both physically and emotionally. Life as a robot was not worth living. However, that goal meant gradually breaking down the powerful repression of those feelings of long ago.

I was committed to her goal. Furthermore, to abandon the ego states with whom I had formed a relationship would prove to them that the world really was harmful and untrustworthy—a reinforcement of the early devastating experiences.

In our work in the fantasied rooms, the Protector learned to relate to the hypnotized Mary, as did the Little Girl. At one session he dared to visit the Little Girl, but he would not touch her for fear that his touch might hurt her. Furthermore, if he touched her it might suggest that he loved her, an emotion that he could not admit. Only much later would they touch.

As for touch, I was very careful with the patient. At the beginning of therapy she warned me not to touch her, and I respected that request. During the second year the Protector and the Little Girl wanted to feel the touch of my hand to see what that felt like. At a much later session I had the Protector touch the Little Girl's hand to see how they both felt. Touch between ego states can be a very effective maneuver to bring ego states closer together.

The therapy was difficult. Sometimes she cried, sometimes she wanted to cry but couldn't. Every time we repeated an abreaction, she felt the somatic pain. She hit walls in frustration, wrote in journals, was conscientious about her psychological homework, and went to work every day. Sometimes I made special audiotapes to which she listened. She worked hard.

As we progressed, the adult Mary began to feel. She liked the ups and downs of emotions. She was surprised she could distinguish between hot and cold in her body. She became more friendly with peers and a bit less serious. Healing was progressing.

Since the Higher Self was an ego state (it had form and function), I asked if he (Mary decided it was male) could help out in the abreaction. The answer was "No." He declared himself as an observer. He could give advice and take her to a scene, but he could not enter the emotions. He was an objective observer, not a participant in emotions.

Mary wrote poignant poems. The following is an example, exactly as she wrote it with no capitals and specific spacing:

> *there is so much pain locked up inside—mummified*
> *encasing rage*
> *locked away my anger has been my prison*
>   *shutting out the world—closing off my senses*
>   *leaving me gray—lifeless*
> *started at two—my father's anger raging against me*
>   *out of control—no way to stop it*
>   *blaming me—my anger*
> *making me promise never to be angry with him again—never*

to push him to violence with my anger
ended at six—my anger raging through me
out of control—no way to stop it
smashing—killing
kittens I had protected and loved
they were helpless
innocent
loving
and my anger killed them
sick with grief—hating myself
I remembered my promise to my father and promised myself I
would never again let the anger out at anything or anyone
outside myself.
So I locked it away and guard it with my life.

How clear she described the encasement of the anger, the self-hate, the origin. No wonder the Protector viewed the anger as a very destructive force that needed to be locked away. The guilt about the kittens had yet to be processed.

Mary began to have problems in her outside world. Her roommate, of whom she was very fond, became distant and less supportive. Her roommate spent more time with another friend. Mary felt rejected. This situation deteriorated until Mary moved to a place of her own. The rejection was difficult for her because it reinforced the learning from her early childhood; namely, that people who are close will abandon her, including all the self-negatives that accompany that thought. During one appointment she brought me her gun for safekeeping, afraid she might use it in a moment of despair.

Although pragmatic events can annoyingly interfere with psychodynamic therapy, it was useful for her to face rejection in the here-and-now with a newfound attitude and behavior. For therapy to be effective, inward change must lead to outward change. Mary expressed her feelings inside my office and expressed increasingly mature behavior on the outside.

Our approach during each weekly session depended on what happened both inwardly and outwardly in the interim between sessions, in addition to the input from the Higher Self and the Protector. The purpose of each session was to continue down the road toward integration and healing—chipping another niche in the fortress.

Her dissociation was so multifold. Pain was separated from the body. Emotions—anger, fear, sadness—were separated from the body, from speech, from thinking. I felt as if I were trying to fit the myriad pieces of a jigsaw puzzle together.

The help of the Higher Self was invaluable. He explained that he came to be when Mary was a baby, so "she might know enough, so she saw the rules." The Higher Self dealt with thinking, with logic, but not with emotions. He was there with information to preserve the system. During therapy he carried out the same function.

The Protector had much to learn, but his learning would come through the emotions. Everything he learned from father was false, yet no one else in Mary's life countered that teaching. Furthermore, the father was a minister, and he said he spoke the word of God. This dogma carried itself into the outside world: Don't speak, don't move, don't feel, don't tell, don't reveal anything, don't be noticed, or you will be hurt. The world is not a safe place. If you love someone, they will hurt you. And if you get hurt, it's your fault. A recipe for depression.

Slowly but persistently, we pressed ever onward. The relationships with the ego states continued, as did the abreactions when indicated.

One abreaction revealed an interesting twist. During the episode when Mary killed the kittens at age 6, the Protector split off the angry part of her, locking it away from consciousness, saying, "How could she hurt those innocent kittens; I played with them. She is too much like Daddy. I had to get rid of her." With dialoguing, the Protector and 6-year-old arrived at a mutual understanding. The Protector understood Mary had to do something with her anger, so she killed the kittens to feel big and strong. "Before that I was little and scared," said the 6-year-old, "then the Protector split me off but he wouldn't be angry at father; he took it out on Mary." The underlying emotion by the Protector was always fear, fear of reprisal by the original father of his memory. The 6-year-old confronted the Protector: "If you attack Mary you're just like father, or just like me when I killed the kittens." That confrontation upset the Protector because he never thought he was expressing anger at Mary but rather containing it. His cutting of Mary, for example, was protective in his mind, not abusive.

We abreacted the scene. The 6-year-old shrank father down to her size and smashed him. The Protector and 6-year-old made peace. It is interesting to note that as the Protector expressed more and more anger, the six-year-old disappeared.

In the abreactive process, after having been rescued by either the Protector or the hypnotized Mary, some temporary ego states, ages 4, 5, and 8, came to live with the 2-year-old. They were not active in the therapy, however, as if in a holding pattern until everything was resolved and integrated.

The primary therapeutic activity involved the hypnotized Mary and the Protector. Mary was understanding and empathic toward the Protector, but also logical in attempting to change his thinking.

Near the end of the second year, following an abreaction, the adult Mary in the waking state said, "That was me!" The dissociation was breaking down. The fortress was eroding.

Her behavior in the world was more self-assertive. For example, she told her boss she was taking off Friday after Thanksgiving—an amazing change for her. She was beginning to ask, "What do *I* want?"

The Protector gradually became more vulnerable and began to feel. He clearly was becoming more of a child. He accused Mary of wanting to take his power away and leave him with bad feelings. She wrote him a letter offering to share feelings and to hold each other. That made a big difference to him. Having the promise written down not to weaken him and not to hurt him intentionally made it real to him. But he was afraid of the process, "because anger protects me from the pain; it makes it go away." He didn't want to take the risk of giving up the anger, which was his protection from the pain of the past.

He became more desperate. He accused me of eventually abandoning him, just like everybody else. I told him the truth. Therapy is temporary, but Mary is forever. His desperation escalated. At one session Mary was very late. She told me that the Protector tried to prevent her from coming. I hypnotized her and talked to the Protector. In very stern words I declared: "The grown-up Mary has the right to fire me. You don't. And if you ever do that again, I will come after her and bring her to the appointment." He knew I meant it, and it never happened again. He had to find out that I was not weak like his mother, that I could be relied upon to do what I said.

In one session I brought my husband (JGW) to talk to the Protector, so that he could meet a male who was not abusive. My husband talked to him about the difference between the Old and New Testament. This session had impact in an unexpected way. The Protector decided that God changed His mind from the Old to the New, from anger to forgiveness and love, and therefore maybe rules could change, after all. Since father represented himself as the voice of God, the two were inseparable in the mind of the Protector. "If Daddy doesn't love me, then God doesn't love me."

The Protector had more to learn. During one session I suggested that he simply watch an abuse experience, and then feel anger and rescue the child. He was surprised to find out that if Mary experienced the anger, she only has to feel it once and then it would be a memory. "You mean I can just be angry and not be little and scared, and if I go back and feel all those things I won't get small and disappear? So it's not that I'm giving my job over to Mary. There will be memories but they don't have to hurt. I like that." Then he became aggressive toward father and threw him against a wall. "Now I can really protect her because I can stop him. I always thought I was feelings in a bowl; now I know I'm the bowl, not what's inside."

The Protector struggled with his relationship with me. On the one hand he wanted me to hug him in fantasy and hold the left hand in reality. (Mary stated the left hand was his; the right was hers.) He believed love was weak and hate was strong. He worried he might hurt me if he released the hate he held. Clearly, he cared about me. He cared about Mary, and so he didn't want her too close. "If you love someone they hurt you. The world is not safe." He found out that he could get angry at Mary, and she still cared. The same was true for me. In the confusion he temporarily walled himself off.

A fantasy trip to the womb was useful. I suggested a warm energy—a cocoon of golden white light surrounding the fetus. The Protector interpreted this experience as follows: "It means I started out good. I don't feel bad about me though sometimes I have bad feelings. So I'm a good person with bad feelings, so I don't have to have them. It's not giving *me* away."

In her own apartment now, the patient reduced her chain smoking to half a pack a day. She started to bike to work. She felt better. She expressed more creativity in her paintings, and lost some of her need to be perfect.

Occasionally the Protector expressed anger at the adult Mary. He wouldn't let her sleep so she might become weak and have less influence on him. Sometimes he shut off her dreams, so upon awakening in panic she wouldn't know why. Impish but fruitless behavior.

The Higher Self suggested the Protector needed to be physically more active and scream out loud. "Fantasy doesn't come into the real world, but sound is in the now, which has impact." Under hypnosis but in reality I gave the Protector a pillow to hit. "I'm moving and making noise. I'm starting to be able to feel it. I know it's me! I know it's me!"

The Protector and the hypnotized Mary became closer. He held my hand and admitted his fears and loneliness, but no longer felt so alone when he touched my hand. I had him feel Mary's hand, so that he would never feel alone again.

Our most poignant session came near the end of therapy. The Protector talked to me while I held his hand: "When I touch her and she starts talking, I get confused. It's time for me to go. She can have the feelings. I need to go away so you can deal with her." His voice began to fade. In a tender voice I told him I cared about him, that he was a wonderful human being who came to protect her. Tears welled up in my eyes. I felt as if he were sacrificing his identity. Then the voice became louder and more clear: "I'm outside the house! I still exist! And I don't have any pain, any bad feelings. I can rest. I can see the house, but I'm on the warm beach. Mary will now have to deal with the house (the fortress) and tear it down. I am good, and I'm not afraid." He was so relieved. It was so strange to him because he never felt so at peace. Upon arousal the patient was amazed, not only because of what the Protector said, but because she saw a little girl in his stead resting on the beach. I interpreted that the Protector wore a male mask because of its belief that only males have strength, and it so desperately needed to appear strong.

The following week Mary brought in a portrait she made of the little girl she once was, sleeping with her two beloved stuffed animals, finally at peace (figure 4). She mused upon the irony of her life: "It's weird to think being bad is to be alive and being good means you're supposed to be dead. I had to be depressed and suicidal so I could stay alive. I needed to know it's okay to be alive and still feel that I'm good."

Ego state treatment was no longer necessary. The fortress had become an empty ruin. The enemy had disappeared a long time ago, and the war was only a memory.

The patient joined a woman's group—women who had been abused who came together to share their experiences. She also saw a career counselor to map out her future. Now she could live in the here and now and leave the past behind. On a couple of occasions I ran into the patient on the street. Two years had passed. She felt fine and reported she had no need to return to therapy.

Addendum

The picture of the little girl, drawn by the patient, sleeping with her stuffed animals, tells it all as a fitting finale to the patient's three-year struggle. No longer beset with pain, fear, and rage, Mary goes her way in the real world as a mature, grown woman forming normal relationships with others and successfully pursuing her chosen career.

Gone is the need for an impenetrable character armor (a fortress) to wall off the anger, the fear, and the pain. This dismantled fortress can no longer warehouse anger that if turned toward her abusing father of long ago, even to the slightest degree, invited immediate, severe pain. That rage, if released, will not now harm others (like the kittens), and if turned inward, impell Mary to self-destruction. Gone are those walls between her and other people, which made her shrink from the slightest intimacies and drove away friends. Missing are the needs to struggle through life feeling as if she were always "bad" and continually blaming herself for the abuse that was heaped upon her as a child. Gone are the compulsions to confront the world with a set of rigid rules: "Don't cry, don't feel, don't complain, be perfect, be obedient, do what you are told, and do it right even if you don't know how." No longer is her ability to love frozen "because loved ones will abandon you" (like mother). And finally, gone is the need of a young state (the Protector) to stubbornly guard the fortress with all its childish concrete thinking, hoping to avoid pain and preserve some small bits of "selfness" that could justify Mary's living.

The Protector is now at peace. Never more need he/she feel abuse from a

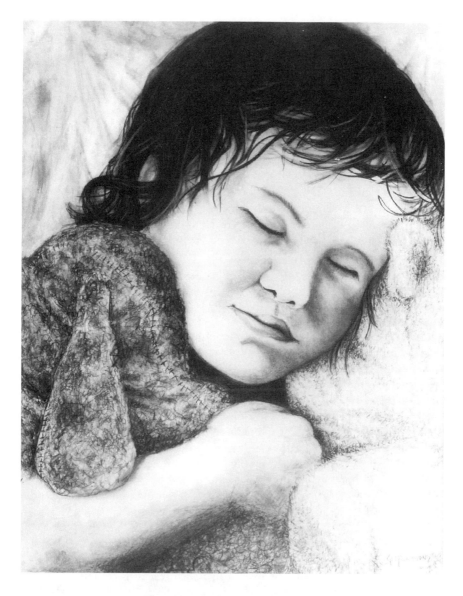

Figure 4. The little girl of long ago.

violent father of the past. The patient can return to her childhood, fully conscious and understanding of it. And now inside Mary, sleeps the little girl with her beloved stuffed animals—as should be the right of all little people in this world.[2]

Some Theoretical Comments (by JGW)

In traditional psychoanalysis the goal is to reconstruct the character structure of the patient so that changes will be long-lasting, not temporary as often occur when symptoms are dismissed through suggestion. Psychoanalytic candidates, after extensive personal analysis, are taught that the development and interpretation of transference reactions, which are then projected onto the analyst, is the truly significant technique for achieving this goal. The good analyst must avoid suggestion, be objective, and passively wait for the appearance of transference behavior by the patient. Appropriate timing of the interpretations is the mark of the experienced clinician. The analyst intervenes with interpretations of resistance or dream material to facilitate the development of these transferences, but otherwise avoids activity.

The goals of full psychoanalysis (involving three to five sessions a week) are usually much more extensive than those that can be achieved in brief (one hour a week) psychotherapy. The aim is complete personality reorganization.

At the termination of a thorough, full, and complete psychoanalysis (usually requiring several hundred hours), the analysand should be able to function symptom-free, have recovered early memories, have achieved insight into and relinquished neurotic defenses, have mastered childhood traumas, be capable of developing good stable object (love) relationships, demonstrate mature behavior in career and interactions with others, and maintain such gains over a long period of time. A thorough, complete character analysis with a difficult case (such as that involving "the Protector") would normally require many hundreds of hours.

By the above criteria the case of "The Protector" would qualify as a full and thorough psychoanalysis. Yet it was accomplished in less than 150 hours of treatment time (once a week for less than three years). How was this possible?

Originally, transference reactions in patients were considered as blocks, contaminants to therapy—and to be avoided. Through incisive observations, Freud and his early associates discovered that such reactions could be turned (through analysis and interpretation) into significant assets toward the achievement of genuine insight—with emotional and experiential components as well as cognitive understanding. A treatment liability was turned into a psychoanalytic asset. The analysis of transference came to be recognized as the most significant therapeutic technique in psychoanalysis. It has remained so for over 80 years.

Unfortunately, waiting for the spontaneous appearance of these reactions and their projection onto the person of the analyst takes much time. Is it possible that some other technique could achieve the same laudable results in much shorter time?

Not only did inappropriate emotions arising in the patient toward the analyst attract the attention of practitioners, but also feelings that were developed in the analyst toward the patient. These were assumed to arise from childhood projections of immature, unresolved problems in the analyst. They were called *countertransferences*. However, these were not turned into therapeutic assets. Rather, they were viewed as blocks and contaminants to the therapy that should be resolved by self or personal analysis of the clinician.

RESONANCE

Not all personal feelings toward the patient arising in the analyst are countertransference; since analysts are human, some feelings may be real. However, there is another source of such feelings. It is called *resonance* (Watkins, J., 1978a).

During resonance the analyst uses his or her entire self (cognitively, affectively, perceptually, and motorically) to develop a replication of the patient, first as object and then by ego cathexis, turning it into a self representation. Now the analyst co-feels, co-pains, co-joys, and co-understands what is present in the self of the patient. He does this with no more than half of his "personhood," while maintaining the other half fully rooted in objective reality (Watkins, J., 1978a).

This is a very powerful technique, allowing the therapist to access a more immediate understanding of the patient's inner psychological situation. Moreover, through counterresonance, the patient rapidly acquires the same meaningful understandings, in his affective, perceptual, motor, and cognitive spheres. Through resonance, the therapist and patient develop a "with-ness," which reassures the patient, allays fears and doubts, and increases emotional strength, thus reducing resistance to interpretations.

Resistances[3] and defenses also lessen in direct proportion to the therapeutic *commitment* of the therapist. The passive, objective analyst commits only the cognitive part of his self. The patient senses this commitment is not total. In resonant ego state therapy the patient unconsciously discerns the much greater commitment (in all spheres) and reacts accordingly. He feels understood in a fuller sense—and hence, loved, since in therapy *understanding equals love*. He does not need his defenses as much. With lowered resistances the treatment proceeds more efficiently, requiring much less time to work through and resolve conflicts.

In Helen's ego state therapy cases, she enters into an intense, resonant relationship with her patients (affectively, perceptually, motorically, *and* cognitively). She uses her whole selfhood as the resonating unit. This brings greater safety to the patient, who then feels understood and not alone. As the intensity of the relationship increases, more therapist activity toward conflict resolution is possible and permissible.

When the therapist, through resonance, takes into her self the patient's problems and coexperiences them in many psychological spheres, the patient reciprocates by coresonating with the therapist and taking back into himself the objective understandings of the clinician—in the same spheres. This constitutes true experiential insight (not only intellectual understanding), which occurs in much less time than in traditional therapy.

In ego state therapy, even interpretations tend to be conveyed through therapist/intra-state behaviors and experiences rather than through verbal-explanatory communications. Following are some examples of ego-state tactics from the Protector case:

- *Page 199* [After a silent abreaction] "[s]he told me she was aware of a Censor inside . . . who determined what she could say and do. . . . Here was the internal replication of the admonitions of her parents." Transference was experienced in the therapeutic hour; it was not projected onto the therapist, but with the ego state "Censor" as the agent and repositor of that transference.
- *Page 200* "My rescuing behavior would have seemed silly at the cognitive, waking level, but we were dealing with hypnotic or unconscious processes. Trance logic is quite different. The past becomes real, as if happening in the present." This therapist activity, therapist rescuing behavior (rather than cognitive interpretation), is made *real* through hypnotic activation. (See Watkins, J., 1954.)
- *Page 201* "Standing up" to experiential mastery of the abuser.
- *Page 202* Frequent experiential abreactions.
- *Page 203* "We struggled together." Resonance.
- *Page 205* "[We] walk down the stairs." Resonance.
- *Page 210* [To the Protector] "if you ever do that again [try to fire the therapist], I will come after her and bring her to the appointment." Therapist activity.
- *Page 211* "In a tender voice I told him I cared about him [the Protector], that he was a wonderful human being who came to protect her. Tears welled up in my eyes. I felt as if he were sacrificing his identity." Resonance, not countertransference.

In summary, good therapy is not so much what we *do to* our patient; it is how we *be with* our patient.

15

TREATMENT OF EARLY TRAUMA AND INSIGHT

Twenty years ago an old maple tree in our front yard died. It was cut down and the stump removed, after which I planted a new young tree, perhaps an inch in diameter. A month later, some child passed by, and with a knife stripped the bark off on one side. Patched up, the little tree survived and grew. It is now fairly large, but the ugly scars on one side are a constant reminder of the early trauma. Such experiences occur to people as well as plants.

When exploring a relatively unknown region, should one stop if approaching a forbidden area? It is much more comfortable to return to safe ground rather than continue when respectable science says, "It's impossible; controlled experimentation has never verified this, etc." We refer here to experiences, that seem to date back to birth or earlier. True, these have seldom been verified in the laboratory as the source of a mental illness or maladaptive behavior, nor that "remembering" them can be curative.

We are also quite familiar with recent research showing in controlled laboratory studies the fallibility of all early memories. That "hypnosis" can elicit as many false or confabulated memories as veridical ones has been demonstrated at statistically significant levels (American Psychiatric Association Board of Trustees, 1994; Bowers & Farvolden, 1996; Frankel, 1994; Garry & Loftus, 1994; Kihlstrom, 1994; Kihlstrom & Evans, 1979; Nash, 1994; Ofshe, 1992; Ofshe & Singer, 1994).

However, other researchers present evidence that hypermnesia (recall of meaningful early events) may be possible, with or without hypnosis (Erdelyi, 1994; Ewen, D., 1994; Nagy, 1994; Spiegel, D., 1991). The pros and cons on the value of recovered memories in therapy has provoked much controversy, especially between researchers and practicing therapists. The literature

217

is too extensive to warrant review here. However, a number of contributors have suggested improvements in clinical practice and approaches toward reconciling experimental and clinical findings (Bloom, 1994a, 1994b; Gravitz, 1994; Lynn, Myers, & Sivec, 1994; Yapko, 1994).

If one only looked at the experimental findings, one would abandon efforts to tap very early experiences as futile. However, even though such early experiences (the first year of life) have not been hypnotically replicated in the laboratory, much observational data in clinical cases indicate that it would be premature to dismiss these possibilities as only "artifacts," "fantasies," "patient expectations," or "reactions to therapist suggestions." Furthermore, if observers only reported findings which agreed with contemporary science and accepted fact, then the discoveries of Copernicus, Galileo, Darwin, Freud, and Einstein would not have enriched the world. Good scientists, while retaining a healthy skepticism, should never say "never" or "impossible." The history of science is full of impossibles becoming possibles and sometimes later verified facts.

Accordingly, with full knowledge that many of our colleagues will disbelieve what we report in this chapter, we would be untrue to our self-view as clinicians and scientists if we failed to present all our data—and perhaps attempted to offer a rationale for them. We refer here to psychological impairments and symptoms reported by some of our patients as "lifelong," and which were resolved (apparently permanently) only when traumatic "experiences," which seemed to have happened in early childhood, and sometimes back to birth (or in utero), were accessed and mastered. We care not whether the modality involved is called hypnosis or guided fantasy or interpersonal relationship. We can only report that in our own scientific skepticism we tried to avoid creating such re-experiencings through therapist suggestions. Sound therapeutic technique must always be, "follow first, then lead," never the other way around. Otherwise, it is the clinician's ideas, theories, and therapy—not the patient's—which prevail.

Those patients who led the treatment into these "preverbal" and perhaps "birth" regions did not get there because the therapist said, "Now we will go back to your birth experience." They occurred indirectly through behaviors, postures, gestures and movements which appeared to be much more than conscious acting. Nor did we hear patients say, "Now I'm being born. I can feel myself coming out the birth canal," etc. We, too, would be rightfully skeptical at such remarks. As our experimental colleagues have frequently pointed out to us, "The child has no language or words at that time. How can a patient speak of such things unless it is sheer fantasy, confabulation, false memory, or acting to please the doctor?" We have consistently tried to remain skeptical and ask ourselves these same questions. But the contrary evidence brought to our attention demands to be reported, common sense or otherwise.

While we know that memories can be partly or entirely false, stemming from fantasies and wishes, we also know that they can be true or partly true (Brown, Scheflin, & Hammond, 1997). If this were not the case, courts should never accept any witnesses' memories into evidence. Nor could this society function if all reported memories must be considered false. While contemporary scientific findings report that memories under hypnosis can not be shown to be superior to those in the conscious state, neither have they proven that hypnotic memories are per se inferior. However, Kihlstrom (1994), who has been in the forefront of researchers that have demonstrated the unreliability of hypnotically recovered memories, concedes that, "It is possible, at least in principle, that hypnosis could be used to structure a hallucinated environment that returns the person to the circumstances, both environmental and emotional, of the forgotten episode: If accurate, this would be the richest retrieval cue imaginable."[1] We leave it to our readers to determine whether the material we present here is compelling evidence of "rich" retrieval or not.

Perhaps the greatest research error is that while experimenters challenge verbal memories, they ignore "memories" communicated nonverbally. Memories are recorded in tissues—even if we cannot observe them. A one-day-old child will experience pain if scalded, even though he or she has no words at that time. At a later age when she has language, she has words that attach to pain. Under hypnosis she may be able to recall the earlier incident and describe or even re-experience it.

As mentioned previously, one of us (HHW) did not speak English as a child, but can report memories in the English language (which was only learned after age 10), for example, recollections of playing around a Bavarian castle at the age of five. This does not involve first thinking of them in German, and then translating them into English words.[2] Images and experiences do not require words to have been recorded.

And if an individual, after acquiring words (stimulus cues to experience) can remember and report the pain of a scalding suffered just after birth, why is it not possible for him or her to have tissue recorded memories of other lesser traumas, discomforts stemming from birth separation, starvation pains from lack of being fed by the mother, or even chemical assaults prebirth?

If a prebirth trauma (physical, genetic, or chemical) results in a visibly deformed child, no one would question a resulting depression, fear, or other psychological dysfunction. It is at least equally possible that less observable trauma resulting from chemical changes caused by maternal rejection could result in psychopathological symptoms and behavior. The problem for the therapist is accessing these areas of experience in the absence of verbal cues attached to them at the time they happened. Our curiosity in this matter was piqued by two unusual therapy sessions that occurred many years ago.

Possible Examples of Very Early Trauma

In a video-recorded therapy session (Watkins, H., 1986a) a college student complained that he always felt "blocked" in whatever he attempted. For example, when he tried to study for an exam he would be blocked, or unable to complete a project. Something seemed to hold him back. He stated that he had suffered this problem all his life.

Helen asked him under hypnosis to "go back to the time [when he] first experienced this blocking." He said nothing but started writhing in his chair, hunching himself forward with slow jerks, finally, much to her surprise, falling partially out of the chair. On coming out of hypnosis he stated that he "felt like being born. It was like being a tiny baby trying to get out." However, he insisted that this couldn't have been a re-experienced birth, because he had been born by cesarean section. At a later session he informed us that he had discussed his birth with his mother, who told him that his birth had been a very difficult and prolonged delivery, but that it had not been a cesarean section.

In a subsequent session, the experience was repeated under deep hypnosis. Only after Helen kept urging him repeatedly with "you can do it; I will help you," did he thrust forward, and with a great spasm, throw himself out completely onto the floor.

During these sessions he would utter no word. Accordingly, the therapist established a form of communication using finger signals (see Cheek, 1962; Rossi & Cheek, 1988). The principle is to inform a mute patient that he can answer questions unconsciously without his awareness by lifting the index finger if the answer would be "yes," the second finger if the answer would be "no," and the third finger if the answer would be "I don't know" or "I don't want to answer." This technique has been used with value by many therapists, including ourselves.

During early sessions, when the patient would writhe in the chair, push forward, but not completely fall out of the chair, he would be asked "Did you do it?" "Are you all the way through?" and he would respond in the negative with a twitching of the second finger. After the final attempt, when he fell completely out of the chair, his index finger lifted, and he indicated a great feeling of relief and ease of breathing. Was this only imagination? However, in subsequent sessions he reported that the lifelong blocking was completely gone, as if he had been completely "reborn" and that the objective of the therapy had been accomplished. He had no further difficulty concentrating and studying, and the blocking did not return.

A colleague of ours, and very experienced physician, on observing the videotape recording of this case (Watkins, H., 1986a), remarked with much excitement that subsequent to the suggestion "to go back to the first time he felt this blocking," the patient assumed the typical fetal position, and that his subsequent movements were also typical of those observed in babies during birth. Is, or is this not, an experiential regression to birth? We have no final verification, but it does raise the question.

The second case, briefly reported earlier (Watkins, J., 1992b), involved a 30-year old woman, an art therapist, who came to HHW for a single appointment. Previously she had had 15 years of therapy, mostly traditional psychoanalysis, and with substantial gain. However, she reported that there was "something missing; something wrong. I keep feeling I am going toward death."

The therapist (HHW), recognizing the futility of asking for a case history (after the patient's 15 years of psychoanalytic therapy), inquired about her birth. She replied that she had been adopted, that her birth mother had been unmarried, and that it was known she had tried to abort her. Helen said, "I suppose she tried to do it with a coat hanger?" Startled, she replied "Why yes, the doctor said I had an injury to my shoulder at birth from the attempt, but how did you know?" Helen pointed to the notepad she was carrying. It was covered with "doodles" in the shape of coat hangers.

She was hypnotized and, using the affect bridge technique, regressed back through time and space to when and where she first felt that feeling (of going to death). Without speaking, the patient lay down on the carpeted floor with knees pulled up. She then scooted herself into a corner of the room.

During this time Helen kept repeating over and over, "You're not supposed to die. You're supposed to live, and you *will* live. I know something is coming after you, but no matter how scary it is, you will live and you're supposed to live!"[3] Finally she slumped in the corner, relaxed. When she was alerted from the hypnosis, the lifelong obsessive feeling of being drawn to death (which had defied 15 years of psychoanalytic therapy) was gone. From later communications she indicated it never returned.

The patient's nonverbal behavior apparently said, "I am about to be destroyed by that thing (object)." Helen's reactions implied, "That is not true. Believe me. You will live. Trust me." The therapist's communications did not involve insight if that is defined as "conscious, cognitive understanding," but it does represent insight if organic meaning is considered, and it was reconstructive of personality functioning.

No believable claim can be made that, if she were regressed to a prebirth level, the fetus could understand Helen's *words*. However, this mastering "re-experience" was carried out in a possibly sensed, accepting, nurturing (mothering) patient-therapist relationship.[4]

When the case was described to a medical colleague, an obstetrician, we were given some *behavioral* confirmation. She informed us that, when an abortion is attempted, the fetus will often try to crawl into the wall of the uterus for safety.

In an effort to understand what happened to these cases in which lifelong impairments, that had resisted years of psychoanalytic treatment, were resolved within a comparatively short period we turned to object-relations theory.

Regression and Object Relations Theory

Object relation theorists have given little consideration to the inner experience of the unborn child except like Fairbairn (1952) and Mahler (1975, 1978) to assume that the child has as yet no internal objects, and that its self is undifferentiated from the mother.

Greenberg and Mitchell (1983, p. 14) define object relations as referring to "individuals' interactions with external and internal (real and imagined) other people, and to relationships between their internal and external object worlds." While most object relations theorists speak of introjects of *people* as internal objects, from the standpoint of Freud's theories, there is no theoretical requirement that the object be a person. Thus, an internal object might stem from the perceived replication of any outside person, thing, or object, with which the self of the individual has interacted in an I-not-I relationship. And as an internal object it may influence thought, feelings, and behavior.

The possibility that object formation may have started prebirth does not seem to have received any attention. Certainly the fetus is in tactual contact with the wall of the uterus, which can expand and contract, even though it adjusts to fetal movements in its softness—thus foreshadowing the later use of a soft *security blanket* as a transitional object.[5]

Other than the impact of chemical changes to maintain homeostasis in the womb, there is minimal (but not entirely absent) stimulation from the outside. It is possible, however, for the fetus to feel tension by an increase of adrenalin from the mother, because adrenalin can pass through the placenta barrier,[6] which is also true of noxious drugs and chemicals. The unborn child apparently can also react to drum rhythms and light and cold (Liley, 1972). Recent British studies (Associated Press, July 6, 1994) have reported that the fetus feels pain in reaction to insertion of a needle for blood transfusion.

Furthermore, the fetus can react to emotional stimuli from the mother (Ferreira, 1965; Sontag & Richards, 1938). Cheek (1975) presented considerable evidence that birth injuries and difficult deliveries can result in imprinted maladjustment patterns, and thus almost certainly the internalization of bad objects.

Watkins, H. (1986b) has recommended expectant mothers to stroke their abdomen and speak reassuring words to the unborn, and especially to sing and "speak" to the fetus. If an abortion is contemplated and deemed necessary, then this behavior is a therapeutic move for the mother.

While Klein (1935) describes how the child "introjects 'good' and 'bad' objects," she assumes that everything that comes from the mother is good and that the bad object represents merely the projection of the child's aggressive drives onto these objects—hence, making them (as she describes) into "persecutors who it fears will devour it, scoop out insides from its body," a threat which Winnicott (1986) characterizes as a more fundamental source of anxiety than castration anxiety or separation anxiety ("It is, in fact, anxiety about annihilation."). Klein, however, insisted that such images are "phantastically distorted pictures of the real object upon which they are based."

She apparently did not conceive of the possible creation of an internal bad object which represented an actual, physical, external bad object, such as a coat hanger by which the mother in Helen's patient attempted to destroy the child. This can hardly be called a mere transitional object which will automatically be dropped in time. Because of the long duration of a sense of impending death in this patient, that had resisted many years of psychoanalysis, it would seem to be a permanent internal object, and the beginning of a *real*, bad object-relationship with the destroying mother (who later abandoned her for adoption). If so, this means that individuation of the fetus, partial development of a self structure, and the establishing of true object relations might possibly begin *before* the time of birth.

In the treatment session the hypnotically regressed infant ego state apparently experienced a transference to the present therapy hour of the original trauma (the coat hanger)—its life threat and damage to her shoulder in the womb—and behaved defensively. Then Helen, by offering a maternal "holding" within that regressed event-in-transference, and by repeating "you are supposed to live" soothingly and confidently, *may* have provided the safety and reassurance, which constituted a "corrective emotional experience," such as described by Alexander and French (1946). The patient reported a new charge of energy, and the fear symptom of impending death disappeared.

Maternal holding or mothering experience appears to be essential in the development of the child if it is to acquire identity and a sense of "selfness." Paul Federn (1952) often used a psychoanalytically trained nurse, Gertrud

Schwing (1954), to provide mothering experience for his schizophrenic patients to supply their infantile lack of it.

The therapeutic experience described here would also be in line with Fairbairn's theory (1952) in which (according to Beckley, 1986, p. 3) "He (Fairbairn) conceives of the psychotherapist as an exorcist who casts out devils (the bad objects) from the unconscious of the patient by providing (herself) as a good object who gives the patient sufficient sense of security to allow the terrifying bad objects to emerge" and be eliminated.

These cases raised questions about the possibility (and validity) of attempts to take therapeutic regressions back into the earliest periods of life, birth, and prebirth. At what point in human development does an individual have the ability to record and be permanently influenced by external stimuli, perhaps noxious ones? And can memories of such be accessed, even though in nonverbal form? Could this be the significant factor in the brief ego state therapies that had succeeded in such comparatively short times?

We decided to study in detail those cases, reported in chapter 13, that had scored the highest success (A +, A, A −) according to the responses on the research questionnaire described in that chapter. What was so different in their treatment that brought outstandingly successful outcomes to those *A* patients who had reported hundreds of hours of psychoanalytic therapy previously with minimal or modest results?

Several of the clients (N = 7), who scored very high, did identify themselves, and thus permitted us to search their case notes for some answer. Every one of these had reported that they had suffered from their problem "lifelong" or the equivalent. In reviewing their records we found that in four out of the seven cases, ego state therapy seemed to reach into early infant, birth, and prebirth trauma areas. In some cases a baby was *seen* as object, that is, as a child state being neglected, starved, or abused by a parent. In two cases the baby was hypnotically experienced as *self* (ego cathected) within the therapy, and interacted with others, often abreacting anger or fear. In all seven cases there were therapeutic regressions prior to the age of three. There was also a crossing back and forth between all age levels, connecting earlier ones with symptoms, feelings, and behaviors at later ages, often with intense abreactions.

Genuine Insight versus Cognitive Insight

Insight has been traditionally considered (Freud, 1938) as a sine qua non for successful therapy. Some researchers, especially those associated with the behavioral school, insist that it is unnecessary and irrelevant in effective therapy. The controversy is a longtime one with pro and con writers publishing many reports (see Bergin & Strupp, 1972). Fisher and Greenberg (1977, see chapter 9) attempted to analyze objective research reports on the ability of insight to effect therapeutic change. They concluded that researchers had largely ignored Freud's concept of "working through," and thus "had not adequately tested Freud's idea of insight."[7]

Hilgard (1987), in his historical review of all psychology in America, classifies psychoanalysis as "psychodynamic, because it is addressed to motivational and emotional conflicts and their resolution," as an "insight therapy, because therapeutic gains are based on an understanding of the influences of recalled experiences from the past upon the present," and as a "depth therapy, because it deals with the unconscious effect on conscious cognition." The key words are "insight," "understanding," and "conscious cognition."

Psychodynamic therapists uniformly seek to achieve insight in their patients, and regard it as very effective. Since experimenters generally reject its necessity, maybe these two groups are understanding and defining the term differently.

The experience we have had with traumas and other malevolent influences, which seem to have been suffered by patients during their earliest periods of life, has suggested to us that perhaps the client's prior work in psychoanalysis (when not completely satisfactory) may have failed to reach far enough back into childhood. Or maybe they had achieved only intellectual insights, (e.g., conscious, cognitive understandings)[8] without affective, perceptual, postural, visceral, and motoric "relivings," in addition to the cognitive ones. In classical psychoanalysis these latter result from "working-through" after initial discovery.

In our ego state therapy abreactions, new understandings were often experienced simultaneously in bursts of global insight. In fact, sometimes the insight was displayed in all the other spheres *except* cognitive. The cases in which the greatest therapeutic outcome and most significant personality changes occurred appeared to be those in which the insight was very broad based.

If the experimentalists' criticism of insight is with the therapy outcomes resulting from *only conscious, cognitive understandings*, then we can agree with them. Perhaps this is the only kind of insight that can be initiated and measured in the laboratory. But therapists who are content with simple "ah-ha" exclamations from their clients have not completed their job. A person is much more than words stemming from the cerebral cortex.

16

DISSOCIATION/INTEGRATION: INTERPERSONAL, INTRAPERSONAL, AND INTERNATIONAL PERSPECTIVES

The study of ego states leaves one with a profound respect for the complexity of humans and the myriad ways in which by taking ourselves apart and putting ourselves together we seek to survive and meet our needs. The search for pleasure, meaning, and above all existence, drives living organisms to incredible feats of organization. In the course of such processes the person adds to and subtracts from his inherent essence, sometimes adaptively and constructively, sometimes maladaptively and destructively. In an ever changing environment that can both nurture and impair, human ingenuity is put to the test as each individual builds a unique "selfhood," a masterpiece of differentiation and integration.

Some people are eminently successful. They put together the patterns of their selves as entities that effectively cope with the vicissitudes of the world in which they exist. They build for long-range goals and erect lives of happiness, meaning, and success. Others, in pitiful efforts to survive harsh or neglecting treatment from those who should have been their caretakers, split themselves into pieces, desperately trying to cope with problems of immediacy, which unfortunately in the long run consign them to chronic lives of pain, misery, and despair.

Human nature is ever hopeful, and new patterns of self-organization are tried. But sometimes the resources available are so inadequate or ineffective that only with outside intervention can the direction of a destructive tide be altered. It is at this point when the need for "helping-others," called therapists, may be essential.

Good therapists, during periods of interpersonal "allyship," accept their patient's struggle as their own, and through a "we-ness" lend what skill and knowledge they possess in a joint rescue endeavor. Sometimes the mutual effort of therapist and patient is successful. The patient emerges with a new perspective, new hope, and new abilities. He or she re-engages the confrontations and influences of the past in the here and now with greater strength and skill, turning past failures into newfound successes. A life that had previously only existed, painfully and meaninglessly, acquires renewed energy in the treatment and completes its destined path with added value to self and fellow humans. Then, we as therapists can rejoice.

Sometimes, however, our best efforts are inadequate. We assist the needing one little or not at all. Our patient's failure is our own, and we too are lessened. It may be that we must then mobilize our own energy resources in a personal struggle to survive as both "persons" and as "helping persons." We must recoup and reintegrate ourselves.

Every therapist who has been confronted with the suicide of a patient knows the sadness and personal pain this brings. But if the therapist cannot resonate with his or her client, co-enjoy and co-suffer the struggles, then he should not be in a helping profession. One must invest of one's self if one is to assist in the rebuilding of another's self.

We are in the business of "self loans." If we are good investors, we are rewarded by sharing in the happiness and achievements of a successful psychotherapy. Our own self and our "therapeutic self" grows. With each success we become stronger, better, and more competent therapists. But with each failure, unless we repair ourselves, we decline. Some clinicians even reach a stage called burnout, where they must devote remaining personal energies to their own survival.

Interpersonal Perspectives

We now know that human "stuff" within individuals is constantly being differentiated and integrated into new units with relative complexity and stability. However, a brief reflection suggests that these same two principles also operate between people as within a single human. Individual persons integrate to form families, organizations, communities, societies, and nations designed to satisfy needs and to promote survival, adaptation, and happiness. Organized group entities are created, divided, and uncreated. Greater complexities are often followed by simplicities and vice versa. Cities, states, and countries are organized to promote better coping with man's environments. The relationships between these are constantly being modified.

Family Ego State Therapy

The family, consisting normally of man, woman, and children, has been tested over the years and found in general to meet many human needs— emotional, personal, sexual, and economic. Yet families often split as the parties involved find themselves incompatible when their frustrations with one another exceed the gratification of their needs within their relationships. Like multiple personalities, they separate and go relatively independent ways.

New integrations, such as single family homes, homosexual ties, etc., are being tried today in the effort to find units that can function effectively and maintain human well-being. Separation, divorce, and remarriage continue to exemplify the principles of differentiation-dissociation and integration.

Within a single individual, psychological geography is all powerful. Ego states must stay together physically because they cannot leave the confines of a single body, thus maintaining a force toward integration, not merely co-existence. In families, the constraints of geography (a jointly owned house) and economics (the necessity of a breadwinner) operate as forces opposing separation. Many couples who are angry and hostile toward one another, who little understand or meet the needs of their spouses, where communication has broken down and emotional walls block off a cooperative relationship, often continue to remain together "for the sake of the children," or because one is dependent on the other for the necessities of life.

Groups, like individuals whose ego states are mutually inimical and non-communicative to one another, may endure neurotic and maladaptive existences, plagued by symptoms and self-defeating behaviors.

If we are to progress in understanding and dealing with human problems, both of individuals and groups, we must acquire new knowledge, new comprehensions how we as people behave and why. Although we learn therapy as a science, we practice it as an art. But the art of psychotherapy must ever be backed by new, scientifically acquired knowledge. We have a few thoughts about research studies that are needed in the field of ego states.

Ego States in Partners

A fruitful and as yet unexplored area in which ego state theory might operate is that of *marital and couples therapy*. At any time one ego state is usually primary, or executive, in an individual. Accordingly, we must assume that the content of the primary state within a husband at a given moment may well determine the type and manner of responses to his wife when they are engaging in mutual activities, such as work, play, making love, child care, vacationing, etc., and that the executive state of the wife then will also influence the activity.

Let us consider a husband, James, who has three primary states, A, B, and C, that alternate in assuming the executive position in his personality. The A state developed as a child, often in interactions with his mother. She was a warm, kindly woman, and the A state experiences women most favorably. The B state developed as he competed with an aggressive younger sister for parental favors. His C state was primarily operative during early school years, when he was with male playmates among whom he was the recognized leader.

Let us now assume that his wife, Edith, has three primary states, F, G, and H. Her F state was built around defenses she developed in coping with an aggressive, abusive father. Her G state had blossomed in early childhood when she visited Grandfather, a man who admired his granddaughter as a wonderful little girl. He constantly appreciated and praised her femininity. Her H state showed itself most clearly when as a student in elementary school she excelled in grades.

Now let us consider how this husband and wife will interact when they are negotiating a vacation plan if the pairing of the executive ego states is his C to her G state. With his C state executive, James views himself as strong, a leader, and the one who is accustomed to making decisions. If Edith's G state is foremost, she will be most agreeable to his decisions, since in transference she may perceive him unconsciously as the present-day embodiment of an admiring grandfather, whom she loved dearly. He may have taken an authoritative role in relation to her grandmother, but in whose presence Edith always felt good. There will probably be no family quarrel at this time in deciding on the vacation, and it will probably reflect James's wishes.

Now let us consider this couple's intimacy in making love, a time in which James's A state ordinarily treats his wife with great affection and consideration. Her G state then might operate to make the pairing a happy one for both spouses. However, if just before or during the experience James's B state emerges, we should expect that his affectionate and sexual feelings might subside as aggressive impulses of hostility and jealousy (a transference from his younger sister) become dominant. The bed encounter then might well develop into a fiasco. Or if Edith's F state takes over, she would no longer perceive him as a loving, older male figure, like grandfather, but as an aggressive, abusive father figure, whom she had often tried to avoid.

The complexity of interpersonal relationships, which cement a marriage in affectionate bonds or destroy it through competitive defenses, can so much depend on how a couple learns to pair respective states in their mutual activities, how they understand the moods of the other, and how they react to a changing ego state climate in the other (Toothman & Phillips, 1996).

Perhaps some day this whole area will be studied, and couples therapy will be modified accordingly. Such ego state counseling might involve the charting (perhaps under hypnosis) of the major patterns in each partner, the times and conditions when any state is generally operative, the reactions that occur under different pairings, etc. From the standpoint of ego state theory couples counseling is a much more complex process than we have considered it in the past.

Ego States and the Law

In the forensic field we do not believe that wrongdoers should be excused simply because they happen to be multiple personalities or because they have no memory of acts carried out by malevolent alters. However, courts, in sentencing, do attempt to determine motivations, whether actions are consciously and willfully planned or the result of temporary lapses in emotional control.

If the concept of multiplicity in all individuals becomes more widely known and accepted, then the effects of covert ego states on behavior might be studied and ascertained by competent court-appointed professionals. Such evaluations could assist in the optimal adjudications of crimes and offenders.

Psychological testing, especially of mental ability, and other psychiatric studies are already accepted in most jurisdictions. However, in view of the great suspicion with which claims of dissociation are perceived by the police and legal professions, we doubt that such measures will be seriously considered in the near future. Multiplicity in humans is not widely understood or accepted by the public in general, and the concept of unconscious processes still activates much opposition, as it did to Freud. People refuse to believe that they are not aware of forces within their own selves, or that they are not complete masters in their own internal self-households.

Physiological Multiplicity

In these past chapters we have focused our attention on the relative psychological multiplicity of the individual person, and the dissociation and integration of his mental segments. "Togetherness" and "apartness" movements seem to typify not only the psychological life of individuals, but also their physiological functioning.

Psychological integration (which we seek to develop in multiple personality patients) involves the intercommunication and cooperation between different parts, or alters. The breaking down or lessening of separating boundaries permits information to reach all aspects of the person and then to organize resources for adaptation and survival. Psychological integration optimizes efficiency in accomplishing these objectives.

Likewise, the human body has a nervous system and other channels of intercommunication between its parts (tissues and organs) designed to optimize adaptation and survival. A lesion in one part of the body, through the sensation of focalized pain, may bring the mobilization of blood circulation,

heart beat, and the immune system. Via intercommunication and cooperation between its parts the entire physiological organism operates to remediate
the situation and assure survival (most of the time). This is physiological or
intrapersonal integration.

Unfortunately, the integration is not perfect or complete. For example,
cancer cells in some organs of the body, such as the colon, prostate, or the
breast in women, may originate and develop, even to the point where
the tumor is no longer treatable without producing pain or otherwise alerting
the other parts of the organism or the entire individual to the danger involved. In other words, they are physiologically dissociated. In such circumstances the understanding and skills of the physician may be severely tested.

Possible Ego State Research

There are other areas in which ego state conceptions may play a significant
role, and which need researching.

1. Memory enhancement is today under much attack, both in experimental and legal circles. Can memories be enhanced if the ego state that was
specifically executive at the time of an experience is reactivated? Experiments
have demonstrated that more veridical memories can be retrieved when the
current emotional state of the subject (mood) is the same as that in which the
material was originally learned (Bower, 1981; Bower, Monteiro, & Gilligan,
1978).[1] The findings on mood retrieval of memories should be applied to ego
states. None of the studies on retrieving memories through hypnosis seem
ever to have considered checking to see if the memories were recovered from
the same ego state that was executive at the time they were learned. Yet
experiments have demonstrated that more, both veridical and confabulated,
recollections are retrieved under hypnosis. Granted, memories can be confabulated and falsified. What is needed now is for solid research to devise ways of
helping subjects to distinguish between the true ones and the confabulated
ones. Surely this is not an unsolvable problem. At least we should be able to
increase the "batting average," so that memories in therapy and in court
could be presented with some probability index. This is the next challenge to
experimentalists in the fields of memory and learning.

2. The finding of Federn (1952, see chapter 2) that psychotic patients can
distinguish between experiences that emanate from internal stimuli and those
whose origins are outside their own selves is a most intriguing one. Both are
experienced as reality, but apparently there is a *qualitative* difference in their
"feel," which enables the hallucinating patient to differentiate reality A experiences (perceptions of the external) from reality B experiences (which originate
from internal stimuli). This finding greatly needs research confirmation or
discarding. If it is true, then the possibility exists that people can *learn* to

discriminate between true memories and confabulated ones, and the whole false memory controversy might become moot. Both therapy and jurisprudence would immeasurably benefit.

3. The possibilities that early life, and even prenatal experiences, might be accessed (as suggested in chapter 15) should not be dismissed. Empirical studies could be undertaken involving the recording of early events by parents and obstetricians, which are then followed up over years of psychological study regarding adjustment and mental health of the individuals involved. Just what are the emotional sequelae of an attempted abortion, or other traumatic experience, to the infant? And what effect do these have on dissociative and integrative processes? Can these early experiences (which are already validated) be recovered in hypnoanalytic or ego state therapy? Today we have mostly questions and a few indirect indicators. Tomorrow we need hard-core answers to such problems. Let us have objective studies by our theorists and researchers, not ridicule. The history of science has always been the opening and exploration of previously unknown (and often disbelieved) areas.

International Perspectives

As we learn more how dissociation and integration are involved in the survival of single persons, can we apply such knowledge to the survival of the human race? Or must we repeat the Civil Wars, the World Wars, and the Vietnams of the past, repetitively splitting our global selves into future Bosnias, Arab-Israeli struggles, and other confrontations of mutual destruction?

The maladjustments of violence and war, in which peoples dissociate from one another, build Berlin walls, fight, kill each other, destroy, and then through peace agreements reintegrate on a national or global scale (witness the American Civil War), seem to parallel what we so often see in the alters of a dissociated individual. Even our enemies in World War II are now our allies. Can we apply our study of ego state behaviors within people to a better comprehension and control of national state-behaviors between peoples—and vice versa?

Why should many vast geographical regions endure as "international multiple personalities?" Perhaps a broad utilization of differentiation-integration understandings on a global scale might bring some new hope. Our diplomats and national leaders could be trained, oriented to act as world-wide therapists in the future, treating and teaching the nation states how to eliminate violent, destructive confrontation and work together. Then perhaps mankind will better survive, meet its needs, and plan for centuries of meaningful future through a healed and integrated "world self."[2]

NOTES

Chapter 1

1. For a comprehensive discussion of dissociation from a historical point of view see Ellenburger, 1970.

Chapter 2

1. The authors believe in complete equality of the sexes. At times, however, we will use the general term "he" or "him" to denote a human being (without sexual identity), thus avoiding the awkwardness that results in frequent repetitions of "he/she," or "him/her."

2. Behaviorists (Watson, 1929) abandoned introspection as a legitimate scientific procedure for acquiring psychological data. They referred to "Comte's Paradox" (see Nelson, 1996) as justification for this rejection. Comte held that it is not possible for an entity to be simultaneously the judge and that which is being judged. Nelson suggested a solution to the problem through "metacognition," or the simultaneous processing by two levels of cognition, the "object level" and the "meta level." However, we feel that the paradox can be resolved more simply if we accept that human beings are relatively dissociated/integrated multiplicities. Introspection then may represent the "observation" of one "part" of the self by another. It thus constitutes a "semi-object" level of observation – not the same entity being simultaneously the perceiver and the perceived. When viewed in this way, introspection becomes a legitimate procedure for gathering data in empirical science, since it involves the observation of one entity by a different one.

3. This change of an ego state from subject to object is humorously portrayed by a Civil War story (Botkin, 1993, p. 543): At the end of the war Congress passed a law requiring Confederate soldiers to take an oath of alle-

233

giance to the Union. A Union General, Benjamin Butler, was presiding at such an occasion when a young Southerner stalled at taking the oath and taunted him saying "We gave you hell at Chickamaugua, General, didn't we?" The General became angry and ordered him to take the oath of allegiance at once or he would be shot. The soldier reluctantly took the oath, looked calmly at the General, then stood up and with great pride proclaimed, "General, I suppose I am a good Yankee and citizen of the United States now?" "I hope so," answered the General. The young man then replied, "Well General, the rebels sure did give us hell at Chickamaugua, didn't they?"

4. A number of years ago a young woman came to therapy complaining about not having "a self." She was a brilliant student. Nevertheless, when an examination paper was returned, she always wondered, "who wrote it?" She had no memory of doing it. She experienced all of her actions as object ("watching somebody else performing them").

5. In recent years a movement termed *self psychology* has developed from the relational wing of object-relations theorists (see Connors, 1994; Goldberg, 1991; Sands, 1989; Ulman & Paul, 1989). Drawing heavily on contributions of Kohut (1977, 1978, 1979), this approach emphasizes the development of self structure, the meaning of events, and the relational interaction between therapist and patient as of greatest importance. Although couched in a different terminology, it points to the same factors that P. Federn (1952) and Weiss (1960) considered significant, and that JGW stressed in his studies in *The Therapeutic Self* (1978a).

6. Some individuals who engage in mental activities requiring much concentration have reported the necessity of taking occasional naps to renew their energies.

7. During World War II, JGW (Watkins, J., 1941) prepared a report and review of the literature on behavioral effects of sleep deprivation as a contribution to the literature on psychological warfare. These involved "mental fatigue, lowered visual acuity, inability to maintain attention, difficulty in equilibrium, increased restlessness, irritability, and a tendency to illusions and hallucinations."

The report was sent to K. M. Dallenbach, Chairman of The Emergency Committee in Psychology, N.R.C., and at the Committee's recommendation forwarded to the U.S. War Department. The findings were supported later by news reports from William A. Shirer's *Berlin Diary* (1941) regarding observed effects of mass bombing on city populations. The report was withheld from publication by request of the British Embassy after study by the British Air Ministry.

8. We do not hold that Federn's two-energy theory is *the* explanation for subject-object and other psychological processes, nor is a belief in it essential for the practice of ego state therapy. Indeed, the very existence of ego and object cathexes awaits future biophysiological research for any confirmation as to their reality. However, among the various personality theories with which we are acquainted, this theory seems to offer the best rationale at the present to account for what happens during psychodynamic transformations.

Chapter 4

1. For other discussions of amnesia see Hilgard, 1977, 1986; Kihlstrom & Evans, 1979; Kirschner, 1973; Loewenstein, 1991; and Schneck, 1948.

2. For a recent comprehensive review of the entire problem see Hammond et al., 1995.

3. MPD is the more traditional abbreviation used for multiple personality disorder, and is widely understood. The psychiatric and psychological professions are currently changing to dissociative identity disorder (DID) as the more recent designation for this condition in the APA's *DSM-IV* (1994). MPD and DID may be considered as referring to the same disorder.

4. Bianchi was accused of killing two girls in Bellingham. Under hypnosis an alter calling itself "Steve" emerged and claimed credit (bragged) about the killings plus others in Los Angeles. At the trial in Bellingham I (JGW) and four other expert witnesses diagnosed him as "insane" with four calling him an MPD or "dissociative reaction" (Watkins, J., 1984). Two diagnosed him as a faking "sociopath" or "antisocial disorder." Bianchi himself insisted, "I'm not a multiple, I'm not crazy, and I didn't kill any girls." He pleaded guilty to two killings in Bellingham and five in Los Angeles, and as part of a plea bargain, agreed to testify against his cousin, Angelo Buono.

In the subsequent Los Angeles trial, the case became highly politicized. One of the professional witnesses changed his diagnosis to "atypical dissociative disorder," which he claimed was due to "the effects of the examining methods themselves." Another witness (see Orne, Dinges, & Orne, 1984) used the Circle-Touch Test to support the claim that Bianchi was faking hypnosis. However, later studies (Eiblmayr, 1987; McConkey, Bryant, Bibb, Kihlstrom, & Tataryn, 1990) reported findings invalidating the criteria on the test Orne quoted in arriving at his "faking" diagnosis. The California judge sided with the minority and dismissed the diagnosis of multiple personality disorder.

I have followed Bianchi in prison for some ten years now, talking to guards and other prison personnel, and to Bianchi himself, several times a year for the last four years. He has no memory of the killings and believes they have convicted the wrong person.

His case was presented in Chicago, November 4, 1994, at the 11th International Conference of Dissociative States together with videotaped excerpts of alter-switching, psychological tests, handwritings, art productions, and diaries. At the end of the presentation the mental health professionals (who were specialists in MPD and dissociation) were asked to write down the diagnosis they would have made to the court. The results were as follows:

sociopath or antisocial personality disorder	3
multiple personality or dissociative identity disorder	85
unable to diagnose	2

At an earlier meeting of mental health professionals (American Society of Clinical Hypnosis workshop, Austin, Texas, October 24, 1994) the same presentation was made with results as follows:

sociopath or antisocial personality disorder	3
multiple personality or dissociative identity disorder	33

The overwhelming number of mental health professionals would apparently have diagnosed him as a true MPD, but the media (PBS) represented him to the public as faking the condition.

Chapter 5

1. Nash (1994) has suggested that veridical insight is not the agent of cure, but rather that "it is the construction of a 'compelling self-narrative' that provides the symptom relief." From this point of view the insight need not necessarily be the uncovering, experiential remembering and reliving of an actual traumatic situation. Rather, an abreactive release of bound affect, followed by a cognitive narrative that "makes sense," veridical or not, would provide the patient with a sufficiently compelling (meaningful) self narrative as to permit relinquishment of symptoms. This position has yet to be tested. Many psychoanalysts would not accept such a formulation as valid, and would maintain that the patient must acquire "genuine," hence veridical, insight to achieve "cure."

During World War II, I (JGW) "altered" the memory of a soldier who was depressed and guilt-ridden because he did not leave his foxhole, which was under fire, to rescue a wounded buddy in "No-Man's Land." When help arrived later the buddy was dead. Under hypnosis, we relived the incident, but at the point where he was "just deciding to go for his buddy regardless of the danger," we visualized his commanding officer arriving and ordering him to "stay under cover" because "I can't afford to lose any more men." His guilt disappeared and the depression lifted, not on the basis of veridical insight, but because of an altered (false) memory suggestively instilled.

My supervisor, a psychoanalyst, dryly remarked, "When you hypnotists get through manipulating patient's memories, we analysts will never be able to straighten them out." I have no follow-up on this case, but people apparently do retain false memories for years (Loftus, 1993), perhaps because of positive reinforcement – in this case the loss of guilt.

2. It should be more fully realized in psychoanalytic circles that hypnosis today is often used by hypnoanalysts in the same way that Freud used dreams – as another "royal road to the unconscious," and it need not necessarily involve "suggestion" – which caused Freud to reject it.

3. In another work (Watkins, J., 1992b, chap. 6) we have detailed many of the dream interpretation techniques that we often use, with and without hypnosis, and some of the ways in which we practiced acquiring skill in them.

4. Federn (1943) advises strongly against interpreting the positive transference of schizophrenics. This often reprecipitates psychotic process. Rather, the positive transference should be maintained to stabilize the relationship with the analyst. Only the negative transferences should be interpreted.

Chapter 6

1. We wish to thank Drs. Jane Harris and Joseph Biron for their contribution to this study.

2. This inability to show a history of dissociation becomes especially important when an MPD alter commits a crime. If dissociation is raised as a defense, the prosecution points out that the defendant had no record of being a multiple in the past. This occurred in the case of Kenneth Bianchi, the "Hillside Strangler" (Watkins, J., 1984).

Chapter 7

1. Anna Freud (1946) used the term "by-passing the ego" (defenses) in criticizing hypnosis and in support of her contention that the therapeutic effects of hypnosis were only temporary, thus justifying its non-use by

analysts. In psychoanalysis a defense would be attacked (consciously) and worked-through, not bypassed, thus permanently eliminating its need.

In hypnoanalysis we may bypass a defense. We also aim at permanently eliminating its need but in a different way. A military analogy might be in order. In the psychoanalytic approach an enemy trench would be stormed and, after much energy expenditure, its ability to resist would be eliminated. The trench would be destroyed. Subsequently, with "insight" the patient abandons it and proceeds toward further therapeutic gains.

Hypnoanalysis might proceed more like present-day military tactics. The defense would be bypassed by paratroopers dropped behind it and attacked from the rear (within the unconscious) perhaps abreactively (but with interpretation), exhausting repressed affect and eliminating its power. The defense thus is discarded by the patient because it is no longer effective. The "ego-loan" in "we-ness" of the intense therapist-patient interpersonal relationship makes this possible. The patient is not devastated but relinquishes the defense, which is no longer tenable. It does not continue to exist (behind the lines, so to speak) repressed and dissociated to arise later and nullify therapeutic gains—as Anna Freud viewed hypnosis. Insights achieved in hypnosis are still made fully conscious. This working-through of the defense is just as permanent as in psychoanalysis.

2. I never transmitted my observations or inferences to the parole board. They might not have been fair. Furthermore, if the parole board believed in my observations and took them into account seriously, the inmates would soon learn about them and change their behavior accordingly. My observations would then invalidate themselves.

3. Member of a group of civic-protesting individuals (so self-termed) who refused to obey laws and challenged the constitutional right of judges and police to have legal jurisdiction over them.

4. HHW was not present during these experiments with her former patients so as not to influence the results.

5. For complete copies of this recording see Watkins and Watkins, 1980.

Chapter 8

1. In another treatise (Watkins, J., 1976) the relationship of resonance to objectivity has been explored in some depth.

2. See chapter 9 for specific examples of the affect bridge and the somatic bridge.

Chapter 9

1. For a much more extensive discussion of abreactions, together with history, literature, theory, and techniques see chapter 4, "Abreactive Techniques," in J. Watkins, 1992b.

2. For a more extensive discussion of this situation see J. Watkins, 1989 and 1993a.

3. A number of writers have cautioned about the danger in abreacting psychotics or near psychotics who do not have enough ego strength to cope with the flood of violent affect released. We recognize this possibility, especially with novices to the field. However, we do believe that in most cases if the therapist resonates enough with the patient (Watkins, J., 1978a), the therapist will not induce the patient to confront more affect than he or she can handle, because when the two are together in a "subjective with-ness" both therapist and patient are stronger. Some therapists avoid abreaction because *they* cannot deal with such severe affects; and if this is true, such therapists are wise in using less aggressive tactics.

In some 40 years with abreactive work by JGW and 20 years by HHW or both of us together, we have not yet seen a case where devastation of the ego occurred because of abreaction, and we have frequently used the tactic. However, we do agree that such a hazard exists if the procedure is used carelessly or without due consideration of the patient's ego strength. The key lies in understanding and resonating with the patient, and not in exceeding one's own experience in initiating these powerful reactions.

4. Note the difference between this hypnoanalytic technique and a psychoanalytic one. In psychoanalysis we would wait passively and patiently for the transfer of the patient's anger toward his dominating father onto the analyst. This might have required many weeks. Through the hypnotic modality, we have reactivated an already established transference onto the commanding officer, revivified it, exhausted the affect that manned its defense, and made the transference interpretation. The entire reaction is just as real and convincing to the patient after emerging from hypnosis as if we had followed the psychoanalytic approach, since it was experienced in the hypnotically activated here and now.

Chapter 10

1. JGW has called this technique "subject-object"(see Watkins, J., 1992b, p. 234).

2. No mysticism is implied here. The internal communication is between

the executive ego state and the object representation of the child—as perceived by the patient.

Chapter 11

1. Space here does not permit the detailing of more such brief cases treated by ego state therapy. However, we have published elsewhere a number of cases treated by this approach in either the weekend marathon format or by a traditional once-a-week frequency (Watkins, H., 1978, 1980b; Watkins, J., 1992b; Watkins & Watkins, 1979, 1981, 1982, 1986, 1990a, 1991, 1993a). We have also often presented audio- or video-recorded verbatim excerpts in our workshops.

Chapter 12

1. Strupp (1996) has noted that, "problems in living that bring patients to psychotherapists are not necessarily 'illness' or 'disorders' (such as those described in *DSM-IV*) for which psychotherapy is prescribed a 'treatment.'" This observation is especially true for those individuals, primarily mental health professionals, who undertook the personal ego state therapy with Helen, which will be described in chapter 13.

2. This result has been called "the do-do bird interpretation" (Newman & Tejeda, 1996), namely that, "all therapies are winners." This finding has been most disconcerting to researchers. To us, it argues that the really significant variables that determine therapy effectiveness may not lie in the specific approach, system, or technique, but may inhere in the applier of a specific approach, hence, the "self" or "personhood" of the therapist. Such a conclusion, of course, would enormously increase the difficulties for scientific investigators. It does support the position of psychoanalysts that the effective training of a therapist requires a *personal analysis*. Of course, the essence may be found to lie in the *interaction* between a given therapist and the specific approach that therapist uses. It suggests at least that significant studies on therapeutic effectiveness require more than expertise in research methodology. These should be undertaken by investigators who are also skilled, sensitive therapists, and who have had much experience treating and working (face-to-face) with live patients that were not merely normal laboratory volunteers. Unfortunately, most therapists don't do research.

3. Belatedly, the importance of the person of the therapist is being recognized as a significant variable (perhaps *the* most important variable) in determining the efficacy of any specific therapeutic approach. See the Spring, 1997, issue of *Clinical Psychology: Science and Practice* with papers by Bergin (1997),

Beutler (1997), Garfield (1997), Lambert and Okiishi (1997), Luborsky, McLellen, Diguier, Woody, and Seligman (1997), Sechrest, McKnight, & McKnight (1996), and Strupp and Anderson (1997).

Chapter 13

1. I (JGW) take full responsibility for this study. Helen was involved only to the extent of furnishing a list of "marathon" patients and addresses and signing the transmittal letter. She did not see the data until after the study had been completed and this chapter written.

2. This explanation and instruction sheet accompanied the questionnaire.

3. These case numbers are not identification numbers of each client. They were assigned to the questionnaires in the order in which they were received back. We wanted each respondent to reply anonymously and thus feel free to report negative or critical results. Accordingly the questionnaires were sent without any identifying sign. Afterward, since many included personal letters or signed comments, we wondered whether this had really been necessary. However, we accepted the loss of further data comparisons with Helen's case notes in favor of client objectivity and candidness.

4. In computing chi-square, the categories "slightly" and "ineffective" were combined to keep expected F from being too small, thus leaving three categories: very effective, somewhat effective, and slightly effective-ineffective.

5. In computing chi-square, the categories "beyond," "exceeded," and "yes" were combined, and "partially," "very little" and "no" were combined. This left three categories: beyond, exceeded, yes; largely; and partially, very little, no.

6. In computing chi-square "slightly effective" and "ineffective" were combined. This left three categories: very effective, somewhat effective, and slightly effective-ineffective.

7. In computing chi-square, "beyond," "exceeded," and "yes" were combined, as were "partially," "very little," and "no." This left three categories: beyond, exceeded, yes; largely; and partially, very little, no.

8. The test-scoring experience of JGW, besides grading student exams and papers for over 50 years as a high school teacher and college professor, included devising and publishing a standardized performance scale (Watkins, J., 1942). He had no knowledge or awareness of the identity of each questionnaire rated.

9. Although item 17 called for comments regarding "it," meaning ego state therapy, some respondents could not resist giving personal reactions to the

therapist, illustrating the difficulty of studying procedures separate from practitioners.

Chapter 14

1. In dealing with an event charged with violent emotions that the patient cannot face at this time, it is often a wise therapeutic move to let her *observe* the event first as object (*it* happened—hallucinated through a one-way vision screen, etc.). After desensitization and ego strengthening she may later be able to actually *experience* the situation in the first person as subject (*I* am there). This is the equivalent of the working-through process in psychoanalysis.

2. In view of the many adult problems stemming from misguided parenting in childhood, we wonder what the world could be like if every child were listened to, understood, and treated with love and respect?

3. We believe that if the passive therapist or analyst offers only a limited and cognitive relationship to the patient, he or she may actually create resistances, which later must be analyzed and worked through.

Chapter 15

1. We assume (as per Kihlstrom, 1994) that there may be a greater potential to tap veridical memories and experiences if through hypnotic regression we approximate the emotional and environmental conditions existing at the time of the targeted incident. Of course, that is exactly at what the affect and somatic bridge techniques aim. In other words, communication is not established verbally but rather through a common experiential matrix, in which organ and "tissue" re-enactments are activated.

2. When visiting her original homeland in Bavaria, Helen finds it much easier to converse freely in German than to do German-English translations while in the U.S. This is because memories and relevant ego states are much easier activated when we return to the environments in which they were first acquired.

3. We must assume that the therapist's manner rather than her exact wording is the reassuring element, since the fetus would not understand words at that time. There is evidence that mothers also communicate with their infants in many other ways than verbal (Cheek, 1996).

4. Is it possible that reconstructive or analytic therapies can reach into preverbal levels and induce corrective emotional experiences if the initiating stimuli were not verbal, but tactual, postural, imaginal, stemming from the

sound of a mothering voice, or the reinstatement of internal behaviors via a somatic bridge? Areas of early conflict might then become available therapeutically that are not currently accessed analytically.

5. When the small child cuddles in a security blanket the warmth and feeling may nonverbally trigger a prebirth memory or even an actual regression to the womb similar to the manner in which an affect bridge operates. Between the two there is a common matrix of feeling.

6. Reported in *Drug and Alcohol Abuse Newsletter*, May, 1978.

7. Another extensive review of research studies bearing on Freud's theories can be found in P. Kline, 1972.

8. Perhaps any therapy that relies almost exclusively on words (verbal cues) to communicate must of necessity have much greater success in activating primarily verbal (cognitive) processes than motor, perceptual, affective, and visceral behaviors as are involved in a total experience, and which do not generally cooperate with one another through words. For example, it is not through words that body tone, heart beat, and adrenal secretions intercommunicate or stimulate one another during a threat to the individual. No wonder so much "insight" is primarily cognitive and intellectual in many therapies. We must never forget that words are only the map, not the territory. They may or may not be gates to the territory of reality (behavior and experience).

Chapter 16

1. By initiating the same mood (depression or elation) the subject experienced when originally learning the material, the investigators may well have also activated the same ego state. However, this matter was never considered or checked—which would have been possible under hypnosis.

2. We consider the foregoing theoretical idealism devoutly to be wished, but the realistic attainment of which today remains doubtful.

REFERENCES

Adams, M. A. (1987). *The internal self helper of persons with multiple personality disorder.* Unpublished master's thesis, State University, Arkansas, The University of Arkansas for Medical Sciences.

Adler, A. (1963). *The practice and theory of individual psychology.* Totowa, NJ: Littlefield, Adams.

Akhatar, S., Lindsey, B., & Kahn, F. W. (1991). Sudden amnesia for personal identity. *Psychosomatic Medicine, 84,* 46–48.

Alexander, F., & French, T. M. (1946). *Psychoanalytic therapy.* New York: Ronald.

Allison, R. B. (1982). Multiple personality and criminal behavior. *American Journal of Forensic Psychiatry, 2,* 32–38.

Allison, R. B. (1984). Difficulties diagnosing the multiple personality syndrome in a death penalty case. *International Journal of Clinical & Experimental Hypnosis, XXXII,* 102–107.

Allison, R. B., & Schwarz, T. (1980). *Minds in many pieces.* New York: Rawson-Wade.

Allport, G. W. (1955). *Becoming: Basic considerations for a psychology of personality.* New Haven, CT: Yale University.

American Psychiatric Association. (1988). Debate by R. Kluft, D. Spiegel, M. Orne, & F. Frankl. *Resolved that multiple personality disorder is a real psychiatric entity.* Washington, DC.

American Psychiatric Association. (1994). *Diagnostic and statistical manual of mental disorders* (4th ed.). Washington, DC: Author.

American Psychiatric Association Board of Trustees. (1994). Statement on memories of sexual abuse. *International Journal of Clinical and Experimental Hypnosis, XLII,* 261–264.

American Psychological Association. (1996). Outcome of psychotherapy. *American Psychologist, 51*(10).

Anderson, G. L. (1992). Dissociation, distress and family function. *Dissociation, V,* 210–215.

Baker, E. L. (1981). A hypnotherapeutic approach to enhance object relatedness in psychotic patients. *International Journal of Clinical and Experimental Hypnosis, 29,* 136–137.

Barlow, D. (1996). Health care policy, psychotherapy research and the future of psychotherapy. *American Psychologist, 51,* 1050–1096.

Beahrs, J. O. (1982). *Unity and multiplicity: Multilevel consciousness of self in hypnosis, psychiatric disorder and mental health*. New York: Brunner/Mazel.

Beahrs, J. O. (1983). Co-consciousness: A common denominator in hypnosis, multiple personality and normality. *American Journal of Clinical Hypnosis, 26*, 100–113.

Beahrs, J. O. (1986). *Limits of scientific psychiatry: The role of uncertainty in mental health*. New York: Brunner/Mazel.

Beck, A. T. (1983). Cognitive theory of depression: New perspectives. In P. J. Clayton & J. E. Barrett (Eds.), *Treatment of depression. Old controversies and new approaches* (pp. 265–290). New York: Raven.

Beckley, P. (Ed.). (1986). *Essential papers on object relations*. New York: New York University.

Bergin, A. E. (1997, Spring). Neglect of the therapist and the human dimensions of change: A commentary. *Clinical Psychology: Science and Practice*, 83–89.

Bergin, A. E., & Lambert, M. J. (1978). The evaluation of therapeutic outcomes. In S. L. Garfield & A. E. Bergin (Eds.), *Handbook of psychotherapy and behavior change*. New York: Wiley.

Bergin, A. E., & Strupp, H. H. (1972). *Changing frontiers in the science of psychotherapy*. Chicago: Aldine-Atherton.

Bernstein, E. M., & Putnam, F. W. (1986). Development, reliability, and validity of a dissociation scale. *Journal of Nervous and Mental Disease, 174*, 727–735.

Beutler, L. E. (1997, Spring). The psychotherapist as a neglected variable in psychotherapy: An illustration by reference to the role of therapist experience and training. *Clinical Psychology: Science and Practice*, 44–52.

Bliss, E. L. (1984). Multiple personalities, related disorders, and hypnosis. *American Journal of Clinical Hypnosis, 7*, 114–123.

Bliss, E. L. (1986). *Multiple personalities, related disorders, and hypnosis*. New York: Oxford University.

Bliss, E. L., Larson, E. M., & Nakashima, S. R. (1983). Auditory hallucinations and schizophrenia. *Journal of Nervous and Mental Disease, 171*, 30–33.

Bloom, P. B. (1994a). Is insight necessary for successful treatment? *American Journal of Clinical Hypnosis, 36*, 172–174.

Bloom, P. B. (1994b). Clinical guidelines in using hypnosis in uncovering memories of sexual abuse: A master class commentary. *International Journal of Clinical and Experimental Hypnosis, XLII*, 173–178.

Boor, M., & Coons, P. (1983). A comprehensive bibliography of literature pertaining to multiple personality. *Psychological Reports, 53*, 295–310.

Botkin, B. A. (1993). *A Civil War treasury of tales, legends, & folklore*. New York: Promontory.

Bower, G. H. (1981). Mood and memory. *American Psychologist, 36*, 129–149.

Bower, G. H., Monteiro, K. P., & Gilligan, S. G. (1978). Emotional mood as a context of learning and recall. *Journal of Verbal Learning and Verbal Behavior, 17*, 573–585.

Bowers, M. K., Brecher-Marer, S., Newton, B. W., Piotrowski, Z., Spyer, T. C., Taylor, W. S., & Watkins, J. G. (1971). The emergence of multiple personalities in the course of hypnotic investigation. *International Journal of Clinical and Experimental Hypnosis, 19*, 57–65.

Bowers, K. S., & Farvolden, P. (1996). Revisiting a century-old Freudian slip—from suggestion disavowed to the truth repressed. *Psychological Bulletin*.

Braun, B. G. (1983). Psychophysiological phenomena in multiple personality and hypnosis. *American Journal of Clinical Hypnosis, 26*, 124–137.

Braun, B. G. (1984). Towards a theory of multiple personality and other dissociative phenomena. *Psychiatric Clinics of North America, 7*, 171–193.

Braun, B. G. (Ed.). (1986). *The treatment of multiple personality disorder.* Washington, DC: American Psychiatric Association.

Braun, B. G. (1988a). The BASK model of dissociation. *Dissociation, I*(1), 4–23.

Braun, B. G. (1988b). The BASK model of dissociation: Part II, Treatment. *Dissociation, I*(2), 16–23.

Brna, T. G., & Wilson, C. C. (1990). Psychogenic amnesia. *American Family Physician, 41*, 229–234.

Brown, D., Scheflin, A. W., & Hammond, D. C. (1997). *Memory, trauma treatment, and the law.* New York: Norton.

Brown, D. P., & Fromm, E. (1986). *Hypnotherapy and hypnoanalysis.* Hillsdale, NJ: Erlbaum.

Buckley, P. (Ed.). (1986). *Essential papers on object relations.* New York: New York University.

Cardeña, E., & Spiegel, D. (1993). Dissociative reactions to the San Francisco Bay area earthquake of 1989. *American Journal of Psychiatry, 150*, 474–478.

Carlson, E. B., & Putnam, F. W. (1993). An update on the Dissociative Experiences Scale. *Dissociation, VI*, 16–27.

Caul, D. (1988). Determining prognosis in the treatment of multiple personality disorder. *Dissociation, II*, 24–26.

Cheek, D. B. (1962). Ideomotor questioning for investigation of subconscious "pain" and target organ vulnerability. *American Journal of Clinical Hypnosis, 5*, 30–41.

Cheek, D. B. (1975). Maladjustment patterns apparently related to imprinting at birth. *American Journal of Clinical Hypnosis, 18*, 75–82.

Cheek, D. B. (1996). Use of the telephone and hypnosis in reversing true preterm labor at 26 weeks: The value of ideomotor questioning in a crisis. *Pre- and Perinatal Psychology Journal, 10*, 273–286.

Christianson, S., & Nilsson, L. (1984). Functional amnesia as induced by a psychological trauma. *Memory and Cognition, 12*, 142–155.

Claghorn, J. L. (1976). *Successful psychotherapy.* New York: Brunner/Mazel.

Comstock, C. (1986, September 20). *The therapeutic utilization of abreactive experiences in the treatment of multiple personality disorder.* Presented at the Third International Conference on Multiple Personalities and Dissociative States, Chicago, IL.

Comstock, C. (1991). The inner self helper and concepts of inner guidance: Historical antecedents, its role within dissociation and clinical utilization. *Dissociation, IV*, 165–177.

Connors, M. E. (1994). Symptom formation: An integrative self-psychological perspective. *Psychoanalytic Psychology, 11*, 509–523.

Consumer Reports. (1995, November). Mental health: Does therapy help? 734–739.

Coons, P. M. (1984). The differential diagnosis of multiple personality: A comprehensive review. In B. G. Braun (Ed.), Symposium on multiple personality. *Psychiatric Clinics of North America, 7*, 51–78.

Coons, P. M. (1986). Dissociative disorders: Diagnosis and treatment. *Indiana Medicine, 79*, 410–415.

Coons, P. M. (1988). Psychophysiologic investigation of multiple personality disorder: A review. *Dissociation, I*, 47–53.

Coons, P. M. (1991). Iatrogenesis and malingering of multiple personality disorder in the forensic evaluation of homicide defendants. *Psychiatric Clinics of North America, 14,* 757–768.

Coons, P. M. (1993). Multiple personality disorder consultation in the public psychiatric sector. In R. P. Kluft & C. G. Fine (Eds.), *Clinical perspectives on multiple personality disorder* (pp. 313–325). Washington, DC: American Psychiatric Press.

Coons, P. M., Bowman, E., & Milstein, V. (1988). Multiple personality disorder: A clinical investigation of 25 cases. *Journal of Nervous and Mental Disease, 176,* 519–527.

Coons, P. M., & Milstein, V. (1992). Psychogenic amnesia: A clinical investigation of 25 cases. *Dissociation, V,* 73–79.

Copeland, D. R. (1986). The application of object relations theory to the hypnotherapy of developmental arrests: The borderline patient. *International Journal of Experimental and Clinical Hypnosis, XXXIV,* 157–168.

Cushman, P. (1990). Why the self is empty. *American Psychologist, 45,* 599–611.

Dawson, P. L. (1990). Understanding skepticism toward multiple personality disorder. *American Journal of Occupational Therapy, 44,* 1048–1050.

Dell, P. F. (1988). Professional skepticism about multiple personality. *Journal of Nervous and Mental Disease, 176,* 528–531.

Dickens, C. (1950). *A tale of two cities.* New York: Modern Library.

Douglass, V. F., & Watkins, J. G. (1994). The relation of spontaneous amnesia, ego states, and hidden observers to post-hypnotically dissociated task interference. *Australian Journal of Clinical and Experimental Hypnosis, 22,* 147–152.

Draijer, N., & Boon, S. (1993). The validation of the Dissociative Experiences Scale against the criterion of the SCID-D using receiver operating characteristics (ROC) analysis. *Dissociation, VI,* 28–37.

Edelstien, M. G. (1982). Ego state therapy in the management of resistance. *American Journal of Clinical Hypnosis, 25,* 15–20.

Eiblmayr, K. (1987). Trance logic and the circle-touch test. *Australian Journal of Clinical and Experimental Hypnosis, 15,* 133–145.

Eisen, M. R. (1989). Return of the repressed: Hypnoanalysis of a case of total amnesia. *International Journal of Clinical and Experimental Hypnosis, XXXVIII,* 107–119.

Ellason, J. W., Ross, C. A., Mayran, L. W., & Sainton, M. A. (1994). Convergent validity of the new form of the DES. *Dissociation, VII,* 101–103.

Ellenberger, H. (1970). *The discovery of the unconscious.* New York: Basic.

Emmerson, G., & Farmer, F. (1996). Ego-state therapy and menstrual migraine. *Australian Journal of Clinical Hypnotherapy and Hypnosis, 17*(1).

Ensink, B. J., & van Otterloo, D. (1989). A validation of the Dissociative Experiences Scale in the Netherlands. *Dissociation, 2,* 221–223.

Erdelyi, M. H. (1994). Hypnotic hypermnesia: The empty set of hypermnesia. *International Journal of Clinical and Experimental Hypnosis, XLII,* 379–390.

Erikson, E. H. (1968). *Identity: Youth and crisis.* New York: Norton.

Ewen, D. M. (1994). Many memories retrieved with hypnosis are accurate. *American Journal of Clinical Hypnosis, 36,* 174–186.

Ewen, R. B. (1980). *An introduction to theories of personality.* New York: Academic Press.

Fahy, T. A. (1988). The diagnosis of multiple personality: A critical review. *British Journal of Psychiatry, 153,* 597–606.

Fairbairn, W. R. D. (1952). *An object relation-relations theory of the personality.* New York: Basic.

Fairbairn, W. R. D. (1963). Synopsis of an object-relations theory of the personality. *International Journal of Psychoanalysis, 44.*

Federn, E. (1960, July). Some clinical remarks on the psychopathology of genocide. *The Psychiatric Quarterly,* 1–12.

Federn, E. (1990). *Witnessing psychoanalysis: From Vienna back to Vienna via Buchenwald and the U.S.A.* New York: Brunner/Mazel.

Federn, P. (1928). Narcissism in the structure of the ego. *International Journal of Psychoanalysis, 9,* 401–419.

Federn, P. (1932). The ego feeling in dreams. *Psychoanalytic Quarterly, 1,* 511–542.

Federn, P. (1943). The psychoanalysis of psychosis. *Psychiatric Quarterly, 17,* 3–19, 246–257, 480–487.

Federn, P. (1947a). Principles of psychotherapy in latent schizophrenia. *American Journal of Psychotherapy, 1,* 129–147.

Federn, P. (1947b). Discussion of J. N. Rosen "The treatment of schizophrenic psychosis by direct analytic therapy." *Psychiatric Quarterly, 21,* 25–28.

Federn, P. (1952). In E. Weiss (Ed.), *Ego psychology and the psychoses.* New York: Basic.

Ferreira, A. J. (1965). Emotional factors in prenatal environment. *Journal of Nervous and Mental Disease, 141,* 108–118.

Finch, J. E. (1990). Trust issues with multiple personality clients. *Journal of Mental Health Counseling, 12,* 99–101.

Fine, C. G. (1989). Treatment errors and iatrogenesis across therapeutic modalities in MPD and allied dissociative disorders. *Dissociation, II,* 77–82.

Fine, C. G. (1993). A tactical integrationist perspective on the treatment of multiple personality disorder. In R. P. Kluft & C. G. Fine (Eds.), *Clinical perspectives on multiple personality disorder* (pp. 135–153). Washington, DC: American Psychiatric Press.

Fisher, W., & Greenberg, R. (1977). *The scientific credibility of Freud's theories and therapy.* New York: Basic.

Frank, J. D. (1979). Thirty years of group psychotherapy. *International Journal of Group Therapy, 4,* 239–312.

Frankel, F. H. (1994). The concept of flashbacks in historical perspective. *International Journal of Clinical and Experimental Hypnosis, XLII,* 321–226.

Franks, C. M. (1983). On conceptional and technical integrity in psychoanalysis and behavior therapy, two fundamentally incompatible systems. In H. Arkowitz & S. B. Messer (Eds.), *Psychoanalysis and behavior therapy: Are they compatible?* New York: Plenum.

Fraser, G. A. (1991). The dissociative table technique: A strategy for working with ego states in dissociative disorders and ego-state therapy. *Dissociation, IV,* 205–213.

Frederick, C. (1993). Pools and wellings: The resolution of refractory intermittent depression with ego-state therapy. *Hypnos, 20,* 221–228.

Frederick, C. (1994). Silent partners: The hypnotherapeutic relationship with non-verbal ego states. *Hypnos, XXI,* 141–149.

Frederick, C. (1996). Functionaries, jannisaries and daemons: A differential approach to the management of malevolent ego states. *Hypnos, XXIII,* 37–47.

Frederick, C., & Kim, S. (1993). Heidi and the little girl: The creation of helpful ego states for the management of performance anxiety. *Hypnos, 20,* 49–58.

Frederick, C., & McNeal, S. (1993). From strength to strength: "Inner strength" with immature ego states. *American Journal of Clinical Hypnosis, 35,* 250–256.

Frederick, C., & Phillips, M. (1995). Decoding mystifying signals: Translating symbolic communications of elusive ego states. *American Journal of Clinical Hypnosis, 38,* 87–96.

French, A. P., & Schechmeister, B. R. (1983). The multiple personality syndrome and criminal defense. *Bulletin of the American Academy of Psychiatry and Law, 11,* 17–25.

Freud, A. (1946). *The ego and the mechanisms of defense.* New York: International Universities Press.

Freud, S. (1905). My views on the part played by sexuality in the aetiology of the neuroses. *Collected papers: Vol. 1* (pp. 272–283). London: Hogarth Press & the Institute of Psycho-Analysis.

Freud, S. (1914). On narcissism: An introduction. *Collected Papers: Vol. II* (pp. 30–59). London: Hogarth.

Freud, S. (1922). The infantile genital organization of the libido: A supplement to the theory of sexuality. *Collected papers: Vol. II* (pp. 244–248). London: Hogarth.

Freud, S. (1923). *The ego and the id.* New York: Norton.

Freud, S. (1938). *A general introduction to psychoanalysis.* New York: Pocket.

Freud, S. (1953). The theme of the three caskets. *Collected Papers: Vol. IV* (pp. 244–256). London: Hogarth.

Freud, S., & Breuer, J. (1953). On the psychical mechanism of hysterical phenomena. In *Collected papers: Vol. 1.* London: Hogarth.

Frischholz, E. J. (1985). The relationship among dissociation, hypnosis, and child abuse in the development of multiple personality disorder. In R. P. Kluft (Ed.), *Childhood antecedents of multiple personality* (pp. 100–126). Washington, DC: American.

Frischholz, E. J., Braun, B. G., Martinez-Taboas, A., Ross, C. A., & Van der Hart, O. (1990). Comment on "Is MPD really rare in Japan?" *Dissociation, 3,* 60–61.

Frischholz, E. J., Braun, B. G., Sachs, R. G., Schwartz, D. R., Lewis, J., Shaeffer, B. A., Westergaard, C., & Pasquotto, M. A. (1991). Construct validity of the Dissociative Experiences Scale (DES): I. The relation between the DES and other self-reports of dissociation. *Dissociation, IV,* 185–188.

Frischholz, E. J., Braun, B. G., Sachs, R. B., Schwartz, D. R., Lewis, J., Shaeffer, D., Westergaard, C., & Pasquotto, J. (1992). Construct validity of the Dissociative Experiences Scale: II. Its relationship to hypnotizability. *American Journal of Clinical Hypnosis, 35,* 145–152.

Fromm, Erik. (1964). *The present human condition.* New York: Holt, Rinehart & Winston.

Fromm, Erika. (1968). Transference and counter-transference in hypnoanalysis. *Psychotherapy, Research and Practice, 16,* 77–84.

Fromm, Erika. (1977). An ego-psychological theory for altered states of consciousness. *International Journal of Clinical and Experimental Hypnosis, 25,* 373–387.

Fromm, Erika. (1984). Theory and practice of hypnoanalysis. In W. C. Wester & A. Smith (Eds.), *Clinical hypnosis: A multidisciplinary approach* (pp. 142–154). New York: Lippincott.

Fromm, Erika, & Nash, M. R. (1997). *Psychoanalysis and hypnoanalysis.* Madison, CT: International Universities.

Fromm, Erika, & Shor, R. E. (Eds.). (1979). *Hypnosis: Developments in research and new perspectives* (rev. 2nd ed.). New York: Aldine.

Gainer, M. J., & Torem, M. S. (1993). Ego-state therapy for self-injurious behavior. *American Journal of Clinical Hypnosis, 35,* 257–266.

Ganaway, G. K. (1995). Hypnosis, childhood trauma, and dissociative identity disorder: Toward an integrative theory. *International Journal of Clinical and Experimental Hypnosis, XLIII*, 127–144.

Garfield, S. L. (1997, Spring). The therapist as a neglected variable in psychotherapy research. *Clinical Psychology: Science and Practice*, 40–43.

Garry, M., & Loftus, E. S. (1994). Pseudo memories without hypnosis. *International Journal of Clinical and Experimental Hypnosis, XLII*, 363–378.

Gill, M., & Rapaport, D. (1942). A case of amnesia and its bearing on the theory of amnesia. *Character and Personality, 11*, 166–172.

Goettman, C., Greaves, G. B., & Coons, P. (1994). *Multiple personality and dissociation, 1791–1992. A complete bibliography* (2nd ed.). Lutherville, MD: Sidron.

Goldberg, A. (Ed.). (1991). *The evolution of self psychology: Progress in self psychology* (Vol. 7). Hillsdale, NJ: Analytic.

Goldberg, F. H. (1996). Psychoanalytic practice and managed care: Comparison of Division 39 and other psychologist survey results. *Psychologist Psychoanalyst, XVI*, 3, 1–5.

Goldfried, M., & Wolfe, B. (1996). Psychotherapy practice and research: Repairing a strained alliance. *American Psychologist, 51*, 1007–1016.

Goodman, L., & Peters, J. (1995). Persecutor alters and ego states: Protectors, friends and allies. *Dissociation, 8*, 91–99.

Gravitz, M. A. (1994). Are the right people being trained to use hypnosis? *American Journal of Clinical Hypnosis, 36*, 179–182.

Greaves, G. B. (1988). Common errors in the treatment of multiple personality disorder. *Dissociation, I*, 61–66.

Greenberg, J. R., & Mitchell, S. A. (1983). *Object relations in psychoanalytic theory.* Cambridge: Harvard University Press.

Greenberg, R. M. (1991). Traumatic origins of multiple personality disorder. *Trauma, 32*, 17–21.

Grinker, R. R., & Spiegel, J. P. (1945). *Men under stress.* Philadelphia: Blakiston.

Gross, L., & Ratner, H. (1989). Dissociative disorder in children of holocaust survivors. *Dissociative Disorders: 1989: Proceedings of the Sixth International Conference on Multiple Personality/Dissociative States*, 27.

Gruenwald, D. (1986). Dissociation: Appearance and meaning. *American Journal of Clinical Hypnosis, 29*, 116–122.

Guntrip, H. (1968). *Schizoid phenomena, object relations and the self.* New York: International Universities.

Guntrip, H. (1971). *Psychoanalytic theory, therapy and the self.* New York: Basic.

Hall, C., & Lindzey, G. (Eds.). (1985). *Theories of personality.* New York: Wiley.

Hall, P., & Steinberg, M. (1994). Systematic assessment of dissociative symptoms and disorders in a private practice setting. *Dissociative disorders: 1994, Proceedings of the 11th International Conference on Dissociative States*, 85.

Hammond, D. C., Garver, R. B., Mutter, D. B., Crasilneck, H. B., Frischholz, E., Gravitz, M. A., Hibler, N. S., Olson, J., Scheflin, A., Spiegel, H., & Wester, W. (1995). *Clinical hypnosis and memory: Guidelines for clinicians and for forensic hypnosis.* Des Plaines, IL: American Society of Clinical Hypnosis.

Hartman, W. (1995). *Ego state therapy with sexually traumatized children.* Pretoria, South Africa: Kagiso.

Hartmann, H. (1939). *Ego psychology and the problem of adaptation.* New York: International Universities.

Hartmann, H. (1964). *Essays on ego psychology: Selected problems in psychoanalytic theory.* New York: International Universities.

Hilgard, E. R. (1977). *Divided consciousness: Multiple controls in human thought and action.* New York: Wiley.

Hilgard, E. R. (1986). *Divided consciousness: Multiple controls in human thought and action* (exp. ed.). New York: Wiley.

Hilgard, E. R. (1987). Multiple personality and dissociation. In *Psychology in America: A historical survey* (pp. 303–315). San Diego: Harcourt.

Hilgard, E. R. (1988). Commentary: Professional skepticism about multiple personality. *Journal of Nervous and Mental Disease, 176,* 352.

Hilgard, E. R. (1992). Dissociation and theories of hypnosis. In Erika Fromm & M. R. Nash (Eds.), *Contemporary hypnosis research* (pp. 69–101). New York: Guilford.

Hilgard, E. R., & Loftus, E. F. (1979). Effective interrogation of the eye-witness. *International Journal of Clinical & Experimental Hypnosis, 27,* 342–357.

Hollon, S. (1996). The efficacy and effectiveness of psychotherapy relative to medications. *American Psychologist, 51,* 1025–1039.

Horney, K. (1950). *Neurosis and human growth.* New York: Norton.

Howard, K., Moras, K., Brill, P., Martinovich, Z., & Lutz, W. (1996). Evaluation of psychotherapy: Efficacy, effectiveness, and patient progress. *American Psychologist, 51,* 1059–1064.

Jacobson, E. (1954). The self and the object world. *Psychoanalytic Study of the Child, 9,* 75–127.

Jacobson, E. (1964). *The self and the object world.* New York: International Universities.

Jacobson, N., & Christensen, A. (1996). Studying the effectiveness of psychotherapy: How well can clinical trials do the job? *American Psychologist, 51,* 1031–1039.

Janet, P. (1907). *The major symptoms of hysteria.* New York: Macmillan.

Janet, P. (1925). *Psychological healing: A historical and clinical study.* New York: Macmillan.

Janoff, P. (1970). *Primal scream: A revolutionary cure for neurosis.* New York: Putnam.

Jung, C. G. (1934). *Modern man in search of a soul.* New York: Harcourt-Brace.

Jung, C. G. (1969). *The collected works of C. G. Jung.* Princeton, NJ: Princeton University.

Kernberg, O. (1976). *Object relations theory and clinical psychoanalysis.* New York: Jason Aronson.

Kihlstrom, J. F. (1994). Hypnosis, delayed recall, and the principles of memory. *International Journal of Clinical and Experimental Hypnosis, XLII,* 337–345.

Kihlstrom, J. F., & Evans, F. J. (1979). *Functional disorders of memory.* Hillsdale, NJ: Lawrence Erlbaum.

Kirschner, L. A. (1973). Dissociative reactions: An historical review and clinical study. *Acta Psychiatrica Scandinavica, 49,* 698–711.

Klein, M. (1932). *The psycho-analysis of children.* London: Hogarth.

Klein, M. (1935). A contribution to the psychogenesis of manic-depressive states. In P. Buckley (Ed.), *Essential papers on object relations* (pp. 40–70). New York: New York University.

Klemperer, E. (1968). *Past ego states emerging under hypnoanalysis.* Springfield, IL: Thomas.

Kline, P. (1972). *Fact and fantasy in Freudian theory.* London: Methuen.

Kluft, R. P. (1984). Multiple personality in childhood. In B. G. Braun (Ed.), *The psychiatric clinics of North America: Symposium on multiple personality* (pp. 121–134). Philadelphia: Saunders.

Kluft, R. P. (1987). An update on multiple personality disorder. *Hospital and Community Psychiatry, 38*, 363–373.

Kluft, R. P. (1988). The phenomenology and treatment of extremely complex multiple personality dissociation. *Dissociation, 1*, 47–58.

Kluft, R. P. (1992). The exploration of controversy: Editorial. *Dissociation, 5*, 125–126.

Kluft, R. P. (1993). Clinical approaches to the integration of personalities. In R. P. Kluft & C. G. Fine (Eds.), *Clinical perspectives on multiple personality disorder* (pp. 101–133). Washington, DC: American Psychiatric Press.

Kluft, R. P. (1994). The treatment of dissociative disorder patients: An overview of discoveries, successes, and failures. *Dissociation, VI*, 87–101.

Kluft, R. P., & Fine, C. G. (1993). *Clinical perspectives on multiple personality disorder.* Washington, DC: American Psychiatric Press.

Knowles, F. W. (1964). Hypnosis in amnesic states: A report of seven cases. *New Zealand Medical Journal, 63*, 100–103.

Koch, S. C. (1985). Belief in multiple personality is the first step in diagnosis. *Clinical Psychiatry News, 12*, 3, 24.

Kohut, H. (1977). *The restoration of the self.* New York: International Universities.

Kohut, H. (1978). *The search for the self* (Vols. 1 & 2). New York: International Universities.

Kohut, H. (1979). The two analyses of Mr. Z. *International Journal of Psycho-analysis, 60*, 3–27.

Kris, E. (1951). Ego psychology and interpretation in psychoanalytic therapy. *Psycho-analytic Quarterly, 20*, 15–31.

Kris, E. (Ed.). (1979). *The selected papers of Ernst Kris.* New Haven: Yale University.

LaCalle, R. M. (1991). The bond of trust and the therapeutic alliance. *Beyond survival, 2*(6), 26.

Lambert, M. L., & Okiishi, J. C. (1997, Spring). The effects of the individual psychotherapist and implications for future research. *Clinical Psychology: Science and Practice, 66*–75.

Landman, J. T., & Dawes, R. M. (1982). Psychotherapy outcome: Smith and Glass's conclusions stand up under scrutiny. *American Psychologist, 37*, 504–516.

Lasky, R. (1982). *Evaluating criminal responsibility in multiple personality and related dissociative disorders: A psychoanalytic consideration.* Springfield, IL: Thomas.

Lewis, D. O., & Bard, J. S. (1991). Multiple personality and forensic issues. *Psychiatric Clinics of North America, 14*, 741–756.

Liley, A. W. (1972). Pre-natal child development. *Delta, 9*, 10–15.

Loewenstein, R. J. (1989). Multiple personality disorder: A continuing challenge. *Psychiatric Review, 2*(2), 1–2.

Loewenstein, R. J. (1991). Psychogenic amnesia and psychogenic fugue: A comprehensive review. In A. Tasman & S. M. Goldfinger (Eds.), *American Psychiatric Press review of psychiatry* (Vol. 10, pp. 189–222). Washington, DC: American Psychiatric Press.

Loftus, E. F. (1979). *Eyewitness testimony.* Cambridge, MA: Harvard University.

Loftus, E. F. (1993). The reality of repressed memories. *American Psychologist, 48*, 518–537.

Luborsky, L. A., McLellen, T., Diguer, L., Woody, G., & Seligman, D. A. (1997, Spring). The psychotherapist matters: Comparison of outcomes across twenty-two therapists and seven patient samples. *Clinical Psychology: Science and Practice*, 53–65.

Lynn, S. J., Myers, B., & Sivec, H. (1994). Psychotherapist's beliefs, repressed memories, abuse, and hypnosis: What have we really learned? *American Journal of Clinical Hypnosis, 36*, 182–187.

Mahler, M. S. (Ed.). (1975). *The selected papers of Margaret Mahler*. New York: Jason Aronson.

Mahler, M. S. (1978). *On human symbiosis and the vicissitudes of individuation*. New York: International Universities.

Malcolm, N. (1996). Fear of flying–the use of ego state therapy–two case studies. *Hypnos, XXII*, 202–205.

Malmo, C. (1991). Ego-state therapy: A model for overcoming childhood trauma. *Hypnos, 28*, 39–44.

Maslow, A. H. (1968). *Toward a psychology of being*. New York: Van Nostrand Reinhold.

Mathews, A., Williamson, D. A., & Fuller, R. D. (1992). Mood-congruent memory in depression: Emotional primary or elaboration. *Journal of Abnorman Psychology, 101*(3), 581–586.

May, R. (1980). *Psychology and the human dilemma*. New York: Norton.

McConkey, K. M., Bryant, R. A., Bibb, B. C., Kihlstrom, J. F., & Tataryn, D. J. (1990). Hypnotically suggested anaesthesia and the circle-touch test: A real-simulating comparison. *British Journal of Experimental and Clinical Hypnosis, 7*, 153–157.

McNeal, S., & Frederick, C. (1993). Inner strength and other techniques for ego strengthening. *American Journal of Clinical Hypnosis, 35*, 170–178.

Michelson, L. K., & Ray, W. J. (1996). *Handbook of dissociation: Theoretical, empirical and clinical perspectives*. New York: Plenum.

Miller, S. D., & Triggiano, P. J. (1992). The physiological investigation of multiple personality disorder: Review and update. *American Journal of Clinical Hypnosis, 35*, 47–61.

Moreno, J. L. (1946). *Psycho-drama*. New York: Random House.

Moyers, B. (1993). *Healing and the mind: The mind body connection* (Video-recorded TV documentary). Ambrose Video.

Murray-Jobsis, J. (1984). Hypnosis with severely disturbed patients. In W. C. Wester & A. H. Smith (Eds.), *Clinical hypnosis: A multidisciplinary approach* (pp. 368–404). Philadelphia: Lippincott.

Mutter, C. B. (1990). Hypnosis with defendants: Does it really work? *American Journal of Clinical Hypnosis, 32*, 257–262.

Nadon, R., D'Eon, J., McConkey, K., Laurance, J., & Campbell, R. (1988). Post-hypnotic amnesia, the hidden observer effect, and duality during hypnotic age regression. *International Journal of Clinical & Experimental Hypnosis, 36*, 19–37.

Nagy, T. F. (1994). Incest memories recalled in hypnosis–A case study: A brief communication. *International Journal of Clinical and Experimental Hypnosis, XLII*, 118–126.

Nash, M. R. (1994). Memory distortion and sexual trauma: The problem of false negatives and false positives. *International Journal of Clinical and Experimental Hypnosis, XLII*, 346–362.

Nelson, T. O. (1996). Conscious and metacognition. *American Psychologist, 51*, 102–116.

Newey, A. B. (1986). Ego state therapy with depression. In M. G. Edelstein & D. Araoz (Eds.), *Hypnosis: Questions and answers* (pp. 197–203). New York: Norton.

Newman, F. L., & Tejeda, M. J. (1996). The need for research that is designed to support decisions in the delivery of mental health services. *American Psychologist, 51*, 1040–1049.

Ofshe, R. J. (1992). Inadvertent hypnosis during interrogation: False confession due to dissociative state: Mis-identified multiple personality and the satanic cult hypothesis. *International Journal of Clinical and Experimental Hypnosis, XL*, 135–156.

Ofshe, R. J., & Singer, M. T. (1994). Recovered-memory therapy and robust repression: Influence and pseudomemories. *International Journal of Clinical and Experimental Hypnosis, XLII*, 391–410.

Ondrovick, J., & Hamilton, D. M. (1990). Credibility of victims diagnosed as multiple personality: A case study. *American Journal of Forensic Psychology, 9*, 13–18.

Orne, T. M. (1984). The use and misuse of hypnosis in court. In W. C. Wester & A. H. Smith (Eds.), *Clinical hypnosis: A multidisciplinary approach*. Philadelphia: Lippincott.

Orne, M. T., Dinges, D. E., & Orne, E. C. (1984). On the differential diagnosis of multiple personality in the forensic context. *International Journal of Clinical and Experimental Hypnosis, XXXII*, 311–341.

Pettinati, H. M. (Ed.). (1988). *Hypnosis and memory*. New York: Guilford.

Phillips, D. W. (1994). Initial development and validation of The Phillips Dissociation Scale (PDS) of the MMPI. *Dissociation, VII*, 92–100.

Phillips, M. (1993). The use of ego-state therapy in the treatment of posttraumatic stress disorder. *American Journal of Clinical Hypnosis, 35*, 241–249.

Phillips, M. (1994, March). *Developing a positive transference "trance" in treating post-traumatic patients*. Presented at the annual meeting of the American Society of Clinical Hypnosis, Philadelphia.

Phillips, M., & Frederick, C. (1995). *Healing the divided self: Clinical and Ericksonian hypnotherapy for post-traumatic and dissociative conditions*. New York: Norton.

Piaget, J. (1963). *The language and thought of the child*. New York: World.

Piaget, J. (1966). *Origins of intelligence*. New York: International Universities.

Prince, M. (1905/1929). *The dissociation of a personality*. New York: Longmans-Green.

Putnam, F. W. (1984). The psychophysiological investigation of multiple personality disorder: A review. *Psychiatric Clinics of North America, 7*, 31–41.

Putnam, F. W. (1985). Multiple personality and related dissociative reaction. *International Medicine, 5*, 13–15.

Putnam, F. W. (1986). The treatment of multiple personality: State of the art. In B. G. Braun (Ed.), *The treatment of multiple personality disorder* (pp. 175–198). Washington, DC: American Psychiatric Press.

Putnam, F. W. (1989). *Diagnosis and treatment of multiple personality disorder*. New York: Guilford.

Putnam, F. W. (1991). Recent research on multiple personality disorder. *Psychiatric Clinics of North America, 14*, 489–502.

Putnam, F. W. (1992). Discussion: Are alter personalities fragments or figments? *Psychoanalytic Inquiry, 12*, 95–111.

Putnam, F. W., Guroff, J. J., Silberman, E. K., Barban, L., & Post, R. M. (1986).

The clinical phenomenology of multiple personality disorder: A review of 100 recent cases. *Journal of Clinical Psychiatry, 47*, 285–293.

Ramonth, S. M. (1985). *Multilevel consciousness in meditation, hypnosis, and directed daydreaming.* Upsalla, Sweden: University of UMEA.

Rank, O. (1950). *Will therapy and truth and reality.* New York: Knopf.

Rappaport, D. (1967). *The collected papers of David Rappaport* (M. Gill, Ed.). New York: Basic.

Reagor, P. A., Kasten, J. D., & Morelli, N. (1992). A checklist for screening dissociative disorders in children and adolescents. *Dissociation, V,* 4–19.

Reich, W. (1949). *Character-analysis* (3rd ed.). New York: Orgone Institute.

Reik, T. (1948). *Listening with the third ear.* New York: Farrar.

Reik, T. (1956). *The search within: The inner experiences of a psychoanalyst.* New York: Grove.

Reik, T. (1957). *Of love and lust.* New York: Farrar, Strauss & Cudahy.

Rogers, C. (1980). *A way of being.* Boston: Houghton Mifflin.

Ross, C. A. (1989). *Multiple personality disorder: Diagnosis, clinical features and treatment.* New York: Wiley.

Ross, C. A. (1991). Epidemiology of multiple personality and dissociation. *Psychiatric Clinics of North America, 14,* 503–517.

Ross, C. A., Heber, S., Norton, G. R., Anderson, D., Anderson, G., & Barchet, P. (1989). The dissociative disorders interview schedule: A structured interview. *Dissociation, 2,* 169–189.

Ross, C. A., & Loewenstein, R. J. (1992). Perspectives on multiple personality disorder [Special issue]. *Psychoanalytic Inquiry, 12,* 112–123.

Ross, C. A., Miller, D. S., Bjornson, L., Reagor, P., Fraser, L., & Anderson, G. (1991). Abuse histories in 102 cases of multiple personality disorder. *Canadian Journal of Psychiatry, 36,* 97–101.

Ross, C. A., Norton, G. R., & Anderson, G. (1988). The dissociative experiences scale: A replication study. *Dissociation, I(3),* 21–22.

Rossi, E. L., & Cheek, D. B. (1988). *Mind-body therapy: Methods of ideodynamic healing in hypnosis.* New York: Norton.

Sanders, B., McRoberts, G., & Tollefson, C. (1989). Childhood stress and dissociation in a college population. *Dissociation, 1,* 17–23.

Sanders, S. (1986). The perceptual alteration scale: A scale measuring dissociation. *American Journal of Clinical Hypnosis, 29,* 95–102.

Sands, S. H. (1989). Eating disorders and female development: A self psychological perspective. In A. Goldberg (Ed.), *Dimensions of self experience: Progress in self psychology* (Vol. 5, pp. 75–103). Hillsdale, NJ: Analytic Press.

Sands, S. H. (1994). What is dissociated? *Dissociation, VII,* 145–152.

Sarbin, T. R. (1995). On the belief that one body may be host to two or more personalities. *International Journal of Clinical and Experimental Hypnosis, XLIII,* 163–183.

Savitz, D. B. (1990). The legal defense of persons with the diagnosis of multiple personality disorder. *Dissociation, 3,* 195–203.

Schneck, J. M. (1948). The hypnotic treatment of a patient with amnesia. *Psychoanalytic Review, 35,* 171–177.

Schreiber, F. R. (1974). *Sybil.* New York: Warner.

Schwarzkopf, N. H. (1992). *The autobiography: It doesn't take a hero* (Written by Peter Petre). New York: Bantam.

Schwing, G. (1954). *A way to the soul of the mentally ill.* New York: International Universities.

Sechrest, L., McKnight, P., & McKnight, K. (1996). Calibration of measures for psychotherapy outcome studies. *American Psychologist, 51,* 1065–1071.

Seligman, M. E. P. (1995). The effectiveness of psychotherapy: The *Consumer Reports* study. *American Psychologist, 50,* 965–974.

Seligman, M. E. P. (1996). Science as an ally of practice. *American Psychologist, 51,* 1072–1079.

Selye, H. (1956). *Stress of life.* New York: McGraw-Hill.

Shirer, W. L. (1941). *Berlin Diary.* New York: Knopf.

Smith, M. L., & Glass, G. V. (1981). Meta-analysis of psychotherapy outcome studies. *American Psychologist, 32,* 752–760.

Sontag, L. W., & Richards, T. W. (1938). Studies in fetal behavior. *Monograph of the Society for Research in Child Development, 3.*

Spiegel, D. (1991). Dissociation and trauma. In A. Tasman & S. M. Goldfinger (Eds.), *American press textbook of psychiatry* (Vol. 10). Washington, DC: American Psychiatric Press.

Spiegel, D. (Ed.). (1993). *Dissociative disorders: A clinical review.* Lutherville, MD: Sidran.

Spiegel, H. (1973). *Manual for hypnotic induction profile: Eye-roll levitation method* (Rev. ed.). New York: Soni Medica.

Stampfl, T. G. (1967). Implosive therapy: The theory, the subhuman analog, the strategy, and the technique. Part I: The theory. In S. G. Armitage (Ed.), *Behavior modification techniques in the treatment of emotional disorders.* Battle Creek, MI: Veterans' Administration.

Steckler, J. (1989, October). A workshop with John and Helen Watkins. *Trauma and Recovery,* 25–26.

Steele, K. H. (1989). A model for abreaction with MPD and other dissociative disorders. *Dissociation, II,* 151–159.

Steinberg, M. (1994). *Structured clinical interview for DSM-IV dissociative disorders (SCID-D)* (Rev. ed.). Washington, DC: American Psychiatric Press.

Steinberg, M. (1995). *Handbook for the assessment of dissociation: A clinical guide.* Washington, DC: American Psychiatric Press.

Stekel, W. (1924). *Peculiarities of behavior* (Vols. 1 & 2). New York: Liveright.

Stekel, W. (1943). *The interpretation of dreams* (Vols. 1 & 2). New York: Liveright.

Stekel, W. (1949). *Compulsion and doubt* (Vols. 1 & 2). New York: Liveright.

Strupp, H. (1996). The tripartite model and the *Consumer Reports* study. *American Psychologist, 51,* 1017–1024.

Strupp, H., & Anderson, T. (1997, Spring). On the limitations of therapy manuals. *Clinical Psychology: Science and Practice,* 76–82.

Sullivan, H. S. (1980). *Concepts of personality development and psychiatric illness.* New York: Brunner/Mazel.

Takahashi, Y. (1990). Is multiple personality really rare in Japan? *Dissociation, 3,* 57–59.

Toothman, D., & Phillips, M. (1996). *Ego-state therapy with couples.* (Unpublished manuscript).

Torem, M. S. (1987). Ego-state therapy for eating disorders. *American Journal of Clinical Hypnosis, 30,* 94–104.

Torem, M. S. (1989). Iatrogenic factors in the perpetuation of splitting and multiplicity. *Dissociation, 2,* 92–98.

Torem, M. S. (1993). Therapeutic writing as a form of ego-state therapy. *American Journal of Clinical Hypnosis, 35*, 267–276.

Turner, S. M., Calhoun, K. S., & Adams, H. E. (1981). *Handbook of clinical behavior therapy*. New York: Wiley-Interscience.

Ulman, R., & Paul, P. (1989). A self psychological theory and approach to treating substance abuse disorders: The "intersubjective absorption" hypothesis. In A. Goldberg (Ed.), *Dimensions of self experience: Progress in self psychology* (Vol. 5, pp. 121–141). Hillsdale, NJ: Analytic.

Van der Hart, O. (1990). Comments on "Is MPD rare in Japan?" *Dissociation, 3*, 66–67.

Van der Hart, O. (1993). Multiple personality disorder in Europe: Impressions. *Dissociation, 6*, 102–118.

Van der Hart, O., & Boon, S. (1990). Contemporary interest in multiple personality disorder and child abuse in the Netherlands. *Dissociation, 3*, 66–67.

Vanderlinden, J., Van Dyck, R., Vandereycken, W., & Vertommen, H. (1991). Dissociative experiences in the general population in Netherlands and Belgium: A study with the dissociative questionnaire (DIS-Q). *Dissociation, 4*, 180–184.

Watkins, H. H. (1978). Ego state therapy. In J. G. Watkins (Ed.), *The therapeutic self* (pp. 360–398). New York: Human Sciences.

Watkins, H. H. (1980a). The silent abreaction. *International Journal of Clinical and Experimental Hypnosis, XXVIII*, 101–113.

Watkins, H. H. (1980b). *II. The woman in black and the lady in white* (Audiotape and transcript). New York: Jeffrey Norton.

Watkins, H. H. (1986a). *The trauma of birth: Abreactive therapy* (Videotape). New York: Irvington.

Watkins, H. H. (1986b, Winter). Treating the trauma of abortion. *Pre- and Peri-Natal Psychology*, 135–143.

Watkins, H. H. (1989, October). Therapist's page. *Many Voices*, 4–5.

Watkins, H. H. (1990a). *Raising self esteem: 1. Safe room and life force. 2. The past and you* (Audiotape). Missoula, MT: Author.

Watkins, H. H. (1990b). Suggestions for raising self-esteem. In D. C. Hammond (Ed.), *Handbook of therapeutic suggestions and metaphors* (pp. 127–130). New York: Norton.

Watkins, H. H. (1990c). Hypnotherapeutic procedures for the reduction of guilt. *Hypnos, XVII*, 227–232.

Watkins, H. H. (1993). Ego state therapy: An overview. *American Journal of Clinical Hypnosis, 35*, 232–240.

Watkins, J. G. (1941). *Impairing enemy industrial production through the psychological planning of air raids designed to maximize disruption of worker morale: Studies in cumulative sleep deprivation*. Unpublished confidential report.

Watkins, J. G. (1942). *Objective Measurement of Instrumental Performance*. Contributions to Education No. 860. New York: Columbia University. T. C. Bureau of Publications.

Watkins, J. G. (1946). The hypnoanalytic location of a lost object. *Journal of Clinical Psychology, 2*, 390–394.

Watkins, J. G. (1947). Antisocial compulsions induced under hypnotic trance. *Journal of Social and Abnormal Psychology, 42*, 256–259.

Watkins, J. G. (1949). *Hypnotherapy of war neuroses*. New York: Ronald.

Watkins, J. G. (1951, Summer). A case of hypnotic trance induced in a resistant subject in spite of active opposition. *British Journal of Medical Hypnotism*, 1–6.

Watkins, J. G. (1952). Projective hypnoanalysis. In L. M. LeCron (Ed.), *Experimental hypnosis* (pp. 442–462). New York: Macmillan.

Watkins, J. G. (1954). Trance and transference. *Journal of Clinical and Experimental Hypnosis, 2,* 284–290.

Watkins, J. G. (1960). *General psychotherapy: An outline and study.* Springfield, IL: Thomas.

Watkins, J. G. (1963a). The psychodynamics of hypnotic induction and termination. In J. M. Schneck (Ed.), *Hypnosis in modern medicine.* (3rd ed., pp. 363–389). Springfield, IL: Thomas.

Watkins, J. G. (1963b). Transference aspects of the hypnotic relationship. In M. V. Kline (Ed.), *Clinical correlations of experimental hypnosis* (pp. 5–24). Springfield, IL: Thomas.

Watkins, J. G. (1967). Hypnosis and consciousness from the standpoint of existentialism. In. M. V. Kline (Ed.), *Psychodynamics and hypnosis* (pp. 15–31). Springfield, IL: Thomas.

Watkins, J. G. (1971). The affect bridge: A hypnoanalytic technique. *International Journal of Clinical and Experimental Hypnosis, 19,* 21–27.

Watkins, J. G. (1972). Antisocial behavior under hypnosis: Possible or impossible? *International Journal of Clinical and Experimental Hypnosis, 20,* 95–100.

Watkins, J. G. (1976, Winter). Ego states and the problem of responsibility: A psychological analysis of the Patty Hearst case. *Journal of Psychiatry and Law,* 471–489.

Watkins, J. G. (1977). The psychodynamic manipulation of ego states in hypnotherapy. In F. Antonelli (Ed.), *Therapy in psychosomatic medicine* (Vol. II, pp. 389–403, Symposia). Rome, Italy.

Watkins, J. G. (1978a). *The therapeutic self.* New York: Human Sciences.

Watkins, J. G. (1978b, Winter). Ego states and the problem of responsibility II: The case of Patricia W. *Journal of Psychiatry and Law,* 519–535.

Watkins, J. G. (1984). The Bianchi ("Hillside Strangler") case: Sociopath or multiple personality? *International Journal of Clinical & Experimental Hypnosis, XXXII,* 67–111.

Watkins, J. G. (1987). *Hypnotherapeutic techniques: Clinical hypnosis* (Vol. 1). New York: Irvington.

Watkins, J. G. (1989). Hypnotic hypermnesia and forensic hypnosis: A cross examination. *American Journal of Clinical Hypnosis, 32,* 71–83.

Watkins, J. G. (1992a, April). Psychoanalyse, hypnoanalyse, ego state therapie: Auf der Suche nach einer effektiven Therapie (translated from the English by Monika Amler). *Hypnose und Kognition, Band 9,* 85–97.

Watkins, J. G. (1992b). *Hypnoanalytic Techniques: Clinical Hypnosis* (Vol. 2). New York: Irvington.

Watkins, J. G. (1993a, Fall). Dealing with the problem of "false memory" in clinic and court. *The Journal of Psychiatry and Law,* 297–317.

Watkins, J. G. (1993b). Foreword. *American Journal of Clinical Hypnosis, 35,* 229–231.

Watkins, J. G. (1995). Hypnotic abreactions in the recovery of traumatic memories. *Newsletter of the International Society for the Study of Dissociation, 13,* 1, 6.

Watkins, J. G., & Johnson, R. J. (1982). *We, the divided self.* New York: Irvington.

Watkins, J. G., & Watkins, H. H. (1978). *Abreactive techniques* (Audiotape). New York: Irvington.

Watkins, J. G., & Watkins, H. H. (1979). The theory and practice of ego state therapy. In H. Grayson (Ed.), *Short-term approaches to psychotherapy* (pp. 176–220). New York: Human Sciences.

Watkins, J. G., & Watkins, H. H. (1979–80). Ego states and hidden observers. *Journal of Altered States of Consciousness, 5*, 3–18.

Watkins, J. G., & Watkins, H. H. (1980). *I. Ego states and hidden observers, II. Ego state therapy: The woman in black and the lady in white* (Audiotape and transcript). New York: Jeffrey Norton.

Watkins, J. G., & Watkins, H. H. (1981). Ego state therapy. In R. J. Corsini (Ed.), *Handbook of innovative psychotherapies* (pp. 252–270). New York: Wiley.

Watkins, J. G., & Watkins, H. H. (1982). Ego state therapy. In L. E. Abt & I. R. Stuart (Eds.), *The newer therapies: A source book* (pp. 137–155). New York: Van Nostrand Reinhold.

Watkins, J. G., & Watkins, H. H. (1984). Hazards to the therapist in the treatment of multiple personalities. *Psychiatric Clinics of North America, 7*, 111–119.

Watkins, J. G., & Watkins, H. H. (1986). Ego states as altered states of consciousness. In B. B. Wolman & M. Ullman (Eds.), *Handbook of states of consciousness* (pp. 133–158). New York: Van Nostrand Reinhold.

Watkins, J. G., & Watkins, H. H. (1988). The management of malevolent ego states in multiple personality disorder. *Dissociation, 1*, 67–72.

Watkins, J. G., & Watkins, H. H. (1990a). Ego-state transferences in the hypnoanalytic treatment of dissociative reactions. In M. L. Fass & D. Brown (Eds.), *Creative mastery in hypnosis and hypnoanalysis: A Festschrift for Erika Fromm* (pp. 255–261). Hillsdale, NJ: Lawrence Erlbaum.

Watkins, J. G., & Watkins, H. H. (1990b). Dissociation and displacement: Where goes "the ouch." *American Journal of Clinical Hypnosis, 33*, 1–10.

Watkins, J. G., & Watkins, H. H. (1991). Hypnosis and ego state therapy. In P. A. Keller & S. R. Heyman (Eds.), *Innovations in Clinical Practice* (pp. 23–37). Sarasota, FL: Professional Resource Exchange.

Watkins, J. G., & Watkins, H. H. (1992). A comparison of "hidden observers", ego states and multiple personalities. In W. Bongartz (Ed.), with V. A. Gheorghiu & B. Bongartz (Co-Eds.), *Hypnosis: 175 Years after Mesmer: Recent Developments in Theory and Application* (pp. 315–321). Konstanz: Universitätsverlag Konstanz GmbH (Reprinted 1992 in *Hypnos, XIX*, 215–221).

Watkins, J. G., & Watkins, H. H. (1993a). Ego state therapy in the treatment of dissociative disorders. In R. P. Kluft & C. G. Fine (Eds.), *Clinical perspectives on multiple personality disorder*. Washington, DC: American Psychiatric Press.

Watkins, J. G., & Watkins, H. H. (1993b). Accessing the relevant areas of personality functioning. *American Journal of Clinical Hypnosis, 35*, 277–284.

Watkins, J. G., & Watkins, H. H. (1996a). Overt-covert dissociation and hypnotic ego state therapy. In W. J. Ray & K. Michelson (Eds.), *Handbook of dissociation* (pp. 431–447). New York: Plenum.

Watkins, J. G., & Watkins, H. H. (1996b). Psychodynamic interactions in overt and covert ego states. In B. Burkhard, B. Trenkle, F. Z. Kinzel, C. Duffner, & A. Lost-Peter (Eds.), *Hypnosis International Monographs 2. Munich lectures on hypnosis and psychotherapy*. Munich: M.E.G.-Stiftung.

Watkins, P. C., Mathews, A., Williamson, D. A., & Fuller, R. D. (1982). Mood-congruent memory in depression: Emotional priming or elaboration. *Journal of Abnormal Psychology, 10*, 581–586.

Watson, J. B. (1929). *Psychology from the standpoint of a behaviorist.* Philadelphia: Lippincott.

Weiss, E. (1960). *The structure and dynamics of the human mind.* New York: Grune & Stratton.

Weiss, E. (1966). Paul Federn (1871–1950): The theory of the psychoses. In F. Alexander, S. Eisenstein, & M. Grotjohn (Eds.), *Psychoanalytic pioneers.* New York: Basic.

Wilbur, C. B. (1984). Multiple personality and child abuse. *The Psychiatric Clinics of North America: Symposium on multiple personality* (pp. 3–7). Philadelphia: Saunders.

Winnicott, D. W. (Ed.). (1958). *Collected papers: Through paediatrics to psycho-analysis.* London: Tavistock.

Winnicott, D. W. (1965). *The maturational process and the facilitation environment.* New York: International Universities.

Winnicott, D. W. (1971). *Playing and reality.* London: Tavistock.

Winnicott, D. W. (1986). Transitional objects and transitional phenomena. In P. Buckley (Ed.), *Essential papers on object relations* (pp. 254–271). New York: New York University.

Wollman, B. B., & Ullman, M. (Eds.). (1986). *Handbook of states of consciousness.* New York: Van Nostrand Reinhold.

Wolpe, J. (1982). *The practice of behavior therapy.* New York: Pergamon.

Wright, J. H., Thase, M. E., Beck, A. T., & Ludgate, J. W. (Eds.). (1993). *Cognitive therapy with inpatients: Developing a cognitive mileau* (pp. 22, 147–152). New York: Guilford.

Yapko, M. D. (1994). Suggestibility and repressed memories of abuse: A survey of psychotherapists' beliefs. *American Journal of Clinical Hypnosis, 36,* 163–171.

INDEX